Shift by Shift

Pediatric Home Nursing Guide for Tracheostomy and G-Tube

Dominique Jones

Contents

PREFACE

In the realm of pediatric home nursing, the care of children with tracheostomies and gastrostomy tubes (G-tubes) stands as a testament to the dedication, skill, and compassion of caregivers. These children, often facing complex medical needs, require not just clinical expertise but also emotional resilience and unwavering support.

"Shift by Shift: Pediatric Home Nursing Guide for Tracheostomy and G-Tube Care" emerges as a comprehensive resource designed to empower nurses, caregivers, and healthcare professionals like myself with the knowledge and tools necessary for providing exceptional care in the home setting. Drawing upon evidence-based practices and real-world experiences, this guide has helped me to succeed in my nursing career and will ultimately delves into the intricacies of tracheostomy and G-tube management, offering step-by-step instructions, troubleshooting tips, and insights into fostering developmental milestones.

The journey of caring for a child with a tracheostomy or G-tube is both challenging and profoundly rewarding. As a nurse, I can attest to that. It is a path that requires continuous learning, adaptability, and a deep understanding of the child's unique needs. This guide aims to be a steadfast companion, providing clarity and confidence as caregivers navigate each shift, ensuring that every child receives the highest standard of care in the comfort of their home.

As you embark on this journey, may this guide serve as a beacon of support, knowledge, and encouragement, illuminating the path to compassionate and competent care for every child entrusted to your care.

Dominique Jones

INTRODUCTION

Welcome to Shift by Shift: Pediatric Home Nursing Guide for Tracheostomy and G-Tube Care. This guide was created with one purpose: to support nurses—especially those new to pediatric home health—in delivering safe, confident, and compassionate care for medically fragile children who live with tracheostomies and gastrostomy (G-) tubes.

Who This Book Is For

This book is designed for home health nurses—RNs, LVNs, and even CNAs—working one-on-one with pediatric patients in home settings. Whether you're a new grad entering the world of private duty nursing or an experienced clinician transitioning to pediatrics, this guide walks you through both the morning and night shift routines, step by step.

You'll find practical tips, skill guides, emergency response plans, and real-life scenarios nurses face every shift. If you've ever walked into a child's room unsure of how the day (or night) will unfold—this book is for you.

I. Why "Shift by Shift"?

Unlike a hospital unit or clinic, home nursing care is often done solo. There's no rapid response team down the hall. You're it. Every shift matters. From opening the suction machine in the morning to flushing the G-tube at night, the little details make all the difference in keeping these children safe, clean, nourished, and loved.

This guide mirrors how nurses naturally work—shift by shift—with routines tailored to the rhythm of the child's day and night. Each chapter breaks down core nursing tasks in a clear, repeatable structure so that you can build confidence and competence with every shift.

II. What's Inside

- ***Morning and Night Shift Routines:*** Hour-by-hour breakdowns of what to expect and how to organize your care.
- ***Step-by-Step Skill Guides:*** Easy-to-follow instructions for trach care, suctioning, tube feedings, site care, and more.
- ***Emergency Protocols:*** What to do when something goes wrong.

- ***Real-World Tips:*** From seasoned pediatric nurses working in homecare.
- ***Family Collaboration:*** How to respect and communicate with caregivers in their homes.
- ***Templates & Tools:*** Documentation tips, supply checklists, and handoff notes.

Whether you're reading this on your first day on the job or years into your nursing journey, thank you. Thank you for choosing to care for these children. Their lives are better—and safer—because of you.

Let's get started.

CHAPTER 1
Understanding Home Nursing for Medically Fragile Children

What Is Pediatric Home Nursing?

Pediatric home nursing provides individualized, skilled care to children with complex medical needs in the comfort of their homes. These patients often require continuous monitoring, respiratory support, and feeding assistance due to chronic conditions, prematurity, or neurological disorders. Home nurses play a vital role in keeping these children safe, stable, and able to live as normal a life as possible outside the hospital.

Unlike hospital care, where a team of nurses and providers are just steps away, homecare nurses work independently, relying on their training, judgment, and close partnership with the child's family.

Your Role as a Home Health Nurse

As a home health nurse, your responsibilities may include:

- Monitoring and recording vital signs
- Providing respiratory care, including trach suctioning and oxygen support
- Managing G-tube feedings and medications
- Delivering hygiene and skin care
- Assessing for signs of infection or distress
- Educating family members and supporting their caregiving role
- Documenting all nursing activities and communicating with the child's care team
- Each child's needs will vary, but one constant remains: you are a key member of the child's lifeline, shift by shift.

Working in a Family's Home

Being in someone's home is different than working in a clinical environment. Here are key considerations:

- ***Respect the space:*** Treat the home as the family's safe space. Keep your area clean and organized.
- ***Build trust:*** Parents are often anxious and tired. Be kind, consistent, and open to their insights. They know their child best.
- ***Professional boundaries:*** Be friendly but professional. Clarify your role and avoid overstepping.
- ***Confidentiality:*** Maintain HIPAA standards and protect the family's privacy at all times.
- ***Be flexible:*** Homes are dynamic. You may be working around siblings, pets, or unexpected events. Adapt while keeping care your top priority.

Safety and Legal Responsibilities

Home nurses must follow their state's scope of practice, agency protocols, and care plans prescribed by the child's physician. Documentation is essential—not just for billing or communication, but as a legal record of your care.

Always be prepared for:

1. Emergencies (blocked trach, oxygen desaturation, tube dislodgment)
2. Equipment failure (malfunctioning suction machine, feeding pump errors)
3. Infection control and hand hygiene in a home environment
4. Knowing when to escalate concerns to your agency or medical team
5. Teamwork in Homecare

Although you may work solo on your shift, you're part of a bigger circle:

- Parents and guardians
- Home health agency nurses and supervisors
- Primary care physicians and specialists
- Therapists (PT/OT/ST)
- Medical supply providers
- Collaborative communication ensures consistent care and better outcomes for the child.

This chapter gives new nurses a solid understanding of the home environment and their unique role in it.

CHAPTER 2
Basic Anatomy & Conditions Requiring Tracheostomy and G-Tube Care

Tracheostomy: Why and When It's Needed

A tracheostomy is a surgically created opening in the neck that provides direct access to the airway. In pediatric patients, it is often placed due to:

- Airway obstruction (e.g., subglottic stenosis, vocal cord paralysis)
- Chronic lung disease (e.g., bronchopulmonary dysplasia in preemies)
- Neurological disorders affecting breathing and secretion control (e.g., cerebral palsy, spinal muscular atrophy)
- Prolonged ventilator dependence
- The trach tube bypasses the nose and mouth, providing a secure airway and often connecting to ventilators or oxygen delivery systems.

Pediatric Airway Anatomy Basics

1. Smaller airways mean secretions and swelling can cause rapid distress
2. Infants are nose-breathers, so oral obstruction can escalate quickly
3. Proper trach sizing and securement are essential to maintaining a clear airway
4. Gastrostomy Tubes: Why and When They're Used
5. G-tubes provide direct access to the stomach through the abdominal wall, allowing for feeding, hydration, and medications.

Common reasons for pediatric G-tubes:

- Failure to thrive or inadequate oral intake
- Neurological impairment preventing safe swallowing
- Congenital anomalies like cleft palate or esophageal atresia
- Chronic conditions needing long-term nutritional support

There are several types of G-tubes:

- PEG tubes (initially placed surgically or endoscopically)
- Low-profile "button" tubes (like Mic-Key or Mini-One)
- GJ tubes (for feeds going to the jejunum instead of the stomach)
- Common Diagnoses in Pediatric Homecare
- Understanding the child's diagnosis gives context for your nursing care.

Some examples include:

- ***Prematurity:*** underdeveloped lungs, feeding issues, apnea
- ***Cerebral Palsy:*** poor muscle tone, aspiration risk, mobility challenges
- ***Spinal Muscular Atrophy (SMA):*** progressive muscle weakness, ventilator dependence
- ***Genetic syndromes (e.g., Trisomy 21, CHARGE syndrome):*** variable airway, cardiac, or GI involvement
- ***Seizure disorders:*** risks related to safety and feeding
- ***Trauma or surgery:*** recovery with short- or long-term medical needs

As a nurse, knowing the "why" behind the trach or G-tube helps you anticipate potential problems and customize your care.

CHAPTER 3
Essential Equipment Overview

Pediatric homecare requires mastery of the equipment that supports the child's breathing, nutrition, and overall comfort. As a nurse, you need to be able to set up, use, troubleshoot, and clean each piece of equipment safely—often while responding quickly in high-stress moments. This chapter outlines the most common equipment used in the homes of children with tracheostomies and G-tubes.

1. Suction Machine

Purpose:

To remove secretions from the tracheostomy tube and airway.

Key Features:

- Portable, often battery-powered
- Tubing connects to a suction catheter
- Pressure settings should be adjusted to pediatric levels (typically 80–120 mmHg)

Nurse Tasks:

- Ensure the machine is charged and working at the start of the shift
- Replace canister and tubing as needed
- Suction only as needed, based on assessment (no "routine" suctioning unless ordered)
- Monitor for clear, thin secretions vs. thick, yellow, or bloody ones

2. Oxygen Delivery Systems

Used For:

Children requiring supplemental oxygen via trach collar, nasal cannula, or ventilator

Types of Systems:

- Oxygen concentrator (plugs into the wall, filters room air)
- Compressed oxygen tanks (for portable backup)
- Humidifier bottle (prevents airway drying with trach collar)

Nurse Tasks:

- Check the liter flow matches the physician's order
- Monitor for O2 desaturation with a pulse oximeter
- Prevent tubing kinks or disconnects
- Refill the distilled water in the humidifier chamber as needed

3. Ambu Bag (Bag-Valve-Mask/BVM)

Purpose:

To manually provide breaths in emergencies or during suctioning.

Key Details:

- Must be at bedside at all times
- Attach to trach connector, not face mask, for ventilated/trached children
- Should be tested each shift for functionality

When to Use:

- During trach changes
- In respiratory distress
- After accidental decannulation

4. Feeding Pump

Used For:

Continuous or bolus G-tube feeding

Popular Models:

- Kangaroo Joey
- Infinity pump

Nurse Tasks:

- Program feed and volume correctly
- Prime tubing to remove air before connecting
- Monitor child for signs of intolerance (vomiting, gagging, bloating)
- Flush tube per protocol before and after feeding/meds

5. Pulse Oximeter

Purpose:

Continuous or spot-check monitoring of oxygen saturation (SpO_2) and pulse

Nurse Tasks:

- Place sensor on toe or finger (rotate sites to avoid skin breakdown)
- Know the child's baseline and alarm parameters
- Respond promptly to desaturations (suction, reposition, check O_2 source)

6. Nebulizer Machine

Used For:

Delivering medications to open airways or thin secretions

Nurse Tasks:

- Administer treatments as ordered
- Clean and dry equipment after use
- Monitor for side effects (increased heart rate, jitteriness)

7. Emergency Go-Bag

Every trached child should have a ready-to-go emergency bag with essentials for suctioning, trach changes, and bagging. It may include:

- Suction catheters
- Spare trach (same size and one size smaller)
- Ambu bag
- Water-soluble lubricant
- Obturator
- G-tube extension sets

- Syringes
- Extra pulse ox probes
- Gloves and masks

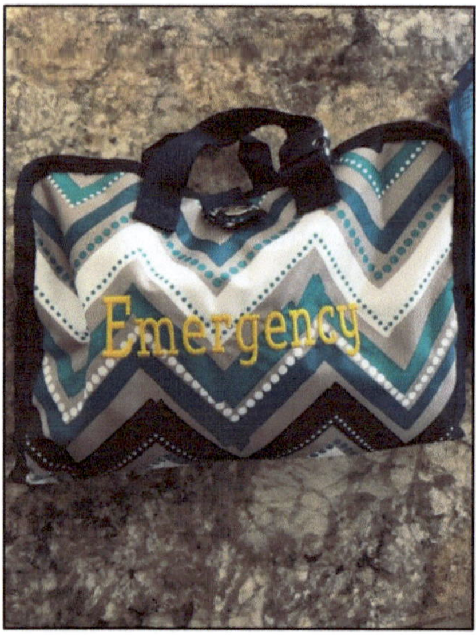

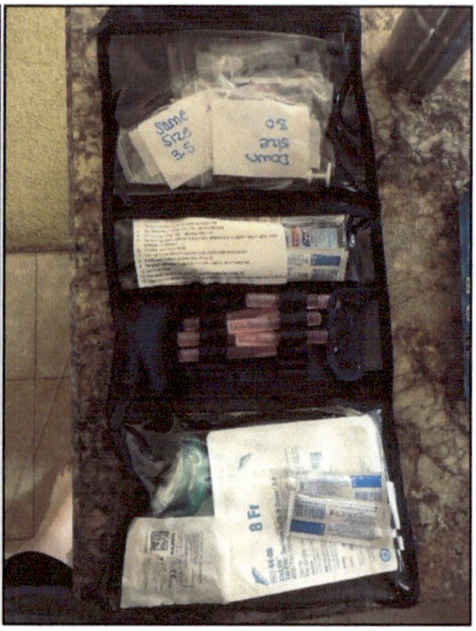

Nurse Tip: Check this bag at the start of every shift. Emergencies happen fast—don't wait until you need it to find out something's missing.

CHAPTER 4
Morning Shift Routine (7 am–3 pm)

A Step-by-Step Guide to Daytime Pediatric Nursing in the Home

The morning shift is where most of the day's structured care happens—feeding, bathing, therapy, medication, and hygiene all center around this part of the day. This is also the shift where the child's schedule overlaps most with family life, school, or in-home therapies.

Start of Shift: Arrival & Assessment

1. Check-in with Parent or Night Nurse (if present):

- Get the handoff report
- Ask about overnight events (e.g., desats, vomiting, sleep patterns)
- Review the care plan and scheduled medications

2. Perform Initial Assessment:

- ***Vital signs:*** heart rate, respiratory rate, temperature, oxygen saturation
- ***Respiratory status:*** listen to lung sounds, check for labored breathing
- ***Skin condition:*** look for rashes, pressure points
- ***G-tube site:*** assess for redness, leakage, granulation
- ***Trach site:*** assess stoma, ties, and tube positioning

3. Prepare Equipment:

- Plug in or test the suction machine
- Ensure oxygen source is working (if applicable)
- Confirm the feeding pump is clean and ready for use
- Restock supplies from the go-bag or home storage
- **8:00–10:00 AM:** Morning Care

4. Trach Care Routine:

- Suction only as needed (signs: coughing, rattling, visible mucus)
- Perform full trach care:
- Wash your hands and wear gloves
- Use sterile cotton-tipped applicators and gauze
- Clean stoma and change ties (per protocol, often every 1–3 days)
- Document appearance and any concerns

5. G-Tube Site Care and Feeding:

- Clean site with warm water and gauze (no alcohol unless ordered)
- Check placement and patency
- Administer a morning bolus or begin continuous feeding
- Flush before and after feed with sterile water or saline
- Document intake and site condition

6. Medication Administration:

- Verify meds with MAR or care plan
- Give via G-tube with proper flushing between meds
- Record time, dosage, and any reactions
- **10:00 AM–12:00 PM:** Personal Care & Development

7. Hygiene and Personal Care:

- Give a full bath (bedside or tub, depending on the child's status)
- Clean behind ears, under neck ties, and under the G-tube dressing
- Perform oral care, even if child is NPO
- Change clothes and diaper or assist with toileting
- Apply lotion or barrier cream as needed

8. Positioning and Mobility:

- Reposition every 2 hours to prevent pressure sores
- Use pillows and supports for comfort and alignment
- Perform a range of motion exercises if indicated
- Support or supervise physical/occupational therapy activities
- **12:00–2:00 PM:** Feeding & Monitoring

9. Midday Feeding and Meds:

- Administer lunch-time G-tube feed
- Give any scheduled noon meds
- Suction or adjust positioning based on respiratory assessment
- Encourage quiet play, tummy time, or time in adaptive equipment

10. Documentation:

- Update charting throughout the shift, including:
- Suctioning events
- G-tube care and feedings
- Medication administration
- Interactions, behaviors, and play
- **2:00–3:00 PM:** End-of-Shift Wrap-Up

11. Final Checks & Communication:

- Reassess vitals and comfort
- Ensure child is clean, fed, and settled for the afternoon
- Update parents on anything important
- Stock supplies and wipe down surfaces

12. Handoff (if PM shift follows):

- Provide a full report:
- Status of trach and G-tube
- Medications given
- Behavioral or clinical concerns
- Any equipment problems
- Leave documentation organized for agency pickup or upload

Shift Tips for Success

- Keep a clipboard with a checklist for tasks and meds
- Ask questions—families are your best resource
- Take mental health moments for yourself during downtime
- Stay alert for subtle changes—small signs can mean big problems in pediatrics

CHAPTER 5
Night Shift Routine (11 pm–7 am)

A Step-by-Step Guide to Overnight Pediatric Nursing in the Home

The night shift is often quieter but still filled with critical tasks. Pediatric home nurses on night shifts must remain vigilant while managing the child's airway, feeding, medications, and safety through a long stretch of hours. It's a time for monitoring and preparation, ensuring the child stays stable until the morning shift.

Start of Shift: Arrival & Initial Assessment

1. Check-in with Parents or Previous Shift Nurse (if present):

Get a detailed handoff report:

- Were there any respiratory issues during the night?
- Any signs of discomfort or distress?
- Review the child's behavior and feeding patterns during the evening
- Review the night care plan for medications and other interventions

2. Perform Initial Assessment:

- ***Vital signs:*** check heart rate, respiratory rate, temperature, oxygen saturation
- ***Respiratory status:*** check for any signs of distress or labored breathing
- ***Skin condition:*** inspect pressure points and any signs of irritation from the G-tube or trach
- ***G-tube site:*** check for leakage, redness, and irritation
- ***Trach site:*** assess the stoma and trach tube for proper placement

3. Prepare Equipment for the Night:

- Ensure that the suction machine, oxygen, pulse oximeter, and feeding pump are ready

- Double-check emergency equipment: ambu bag, spare trach, and go-bag
- **11:30 PM–1:00 AM:** Early Night Care

4. Trach Care Routine:

Perform suctioning as needed (depending on secretions). Full trach care:

- Check the condition of trach ties and change if necessary
- Clean the stoma and tube with sterile cotton swabs or gauze
- Check for signs of infection or blockage
- Record the condition of the airway and any suctioning done

5. G-Tube Care and Feeding:

- Check the G-tube site for irritation, redness, or leakage
- Perform a feed (bolus or continuous as ordered)
- Flush the G-tube with sterile water or saline before and after feeding
- Monitor for any signs of intolerance (e.g., bloating, gagging)
- **1:00 AM–3:00 AM:** Monitoring and Comfort Care

6. Medication Administration:

- Give any scheduled medications as directed, ensuring proper administration through the G-tube
- Flush the G-tube thoroughly between medications
- Keep track of timing and any reactions (alert family if any issues arise)

7. Comfort and Repositioning:

- Reposition every 2 hours to prevent pressure sores
- Use soft supports and pillows for comfort
- Monitor for any discomfort, restlessness, or signs of aspiration
- Check for signs of distress or sudden changes in behavior
- **3:00 AM–5:00 AM:** Ongoing Monitoring & Routine Care

8. Recheck Vital Signs:

- Measure heart rate, respiratory rate, and oxygen levels again

- Watch for any changes in the child's respiratory effort or level of consciousness
- Use the pulse oximeter to check oxygen saturation and make adjustments to O2 as needed

9. Quiet Time & Behavior Monitoring:

- Watch for any signs of discomfort during the night (e.g., grimacing, increased secretions, signs of distress)
- Keep the environment quiet to allow for sleep and recovery
- Provide comfort measures as needed, such as a gentle touch or soft lullabies
- **5:00 AM–6:30 AM:** Preparing for Morning Shift

10. Prepare for Morning Handoff:

Assess the child's status for the incoming shift:

- Is the child stable? Are they comfortable?
- Is the trach clean and secure?
- Was the G-tube feed completed without issues?
- Ensure all equipment is functioning and clean
- Document any observations and make sure all charting is complete

11. Parent Communication (if needed):

- If there are concerns or changes, let parents know so they can prepare for the morning
- Discuss any emergency measures that may need to be in place for the next shift
- **6:30 AM–7:00 AM:** Final Check and Shift Handoff

12. Final Checks:

- Recheck all equipment (e.g., suction machine, O2)
- Ensure the child is comfortable, stable, and in a safe position for the night
- Check that the child's vital signs remain stable

13. Handoff to Morning Shift (if applicable):

- Provide the nurse (or family) with a clear and concise report:
- Respiratory status and any suctioning done
- G-tube and trach care completed
- Medications given and any unusual findings
- Any concerns for the morning shift to watch

Shift Tips for Success

- ***Keep track of time:*** the night shift can be long, but staying on top of tasks helps ensure nothing is missed
- ***Respond to alarms promptly:*** a desaturation or feeding pump issue can escalate quickly
- ***Stay alert to changes in breathing:*** children with trachs can have sudden airway changes, especially at night
- ***Take care of yourself:*** staying rested during the day is critical to maintaining focus during long shifts

CHAPTER 6
Tracheostomy Care

Detailed Guide to Trach Care, Suctioning, and Emergencies

Tracheostomy care is a critical part of pediatric home nursing. The child's trach tube serves as their airway, and any problems with it can quickly become life-threatening. Understanding how to properly care for, monitor, and respond to issues with the trach is essential for your success as a home health nurse.

1. Trach Care Basics: Key Principles

Importance of Tracheostomy Care:

A trach tube bypasses the child's normal upper airway defenses, so the trachea is more prone to infection, irritation, and obstruction. Keeping the tube clean, clear, and secure is vital to ensure the child can breathe easily.

Tracheostomy Care Supplies:

- Sterile gloves
- Gauze pads
- Sterile saline or water for cleaning
- Trach tube ties (or velcro-style ties)
- Cotton-tipped applicators
- Trach dressing (if used)
- Obturator (for emergency reintubation)
- Extra trach tube (same size and one size smaller)
- Suction equipment

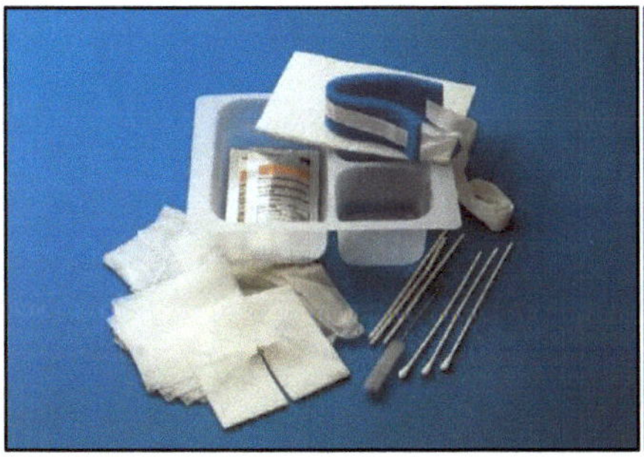

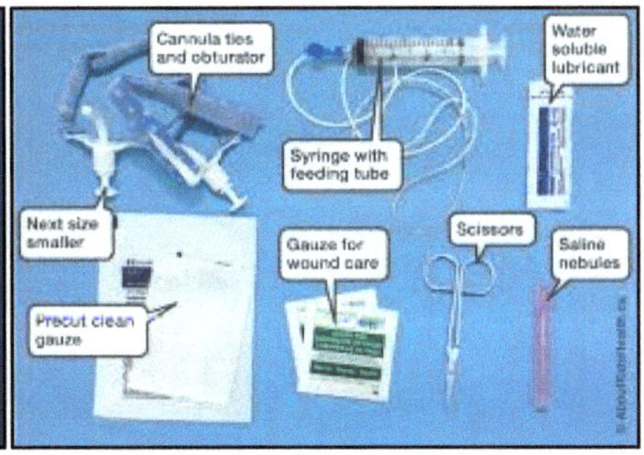

2. Suctioning the Tracheostomy Tube

Why Suctioning Is Needed:

Suctioning removes mucus and other secretions from the child's trach tube and airway. Failure to suction regularly can lead to airway obstruction, respiratory distress, and infection.

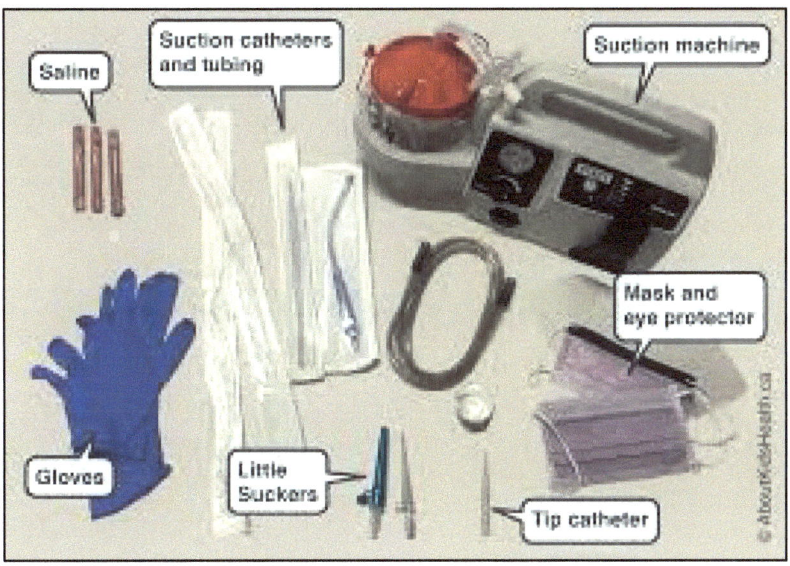

Signs a Child Needs Suctioning:

- Coughing or gagging
- Rattling or gurgling sounds when breathing
- Decreased oxygen saturation (SpO_2)
- Visible mucus in the trach tube or around the stoma

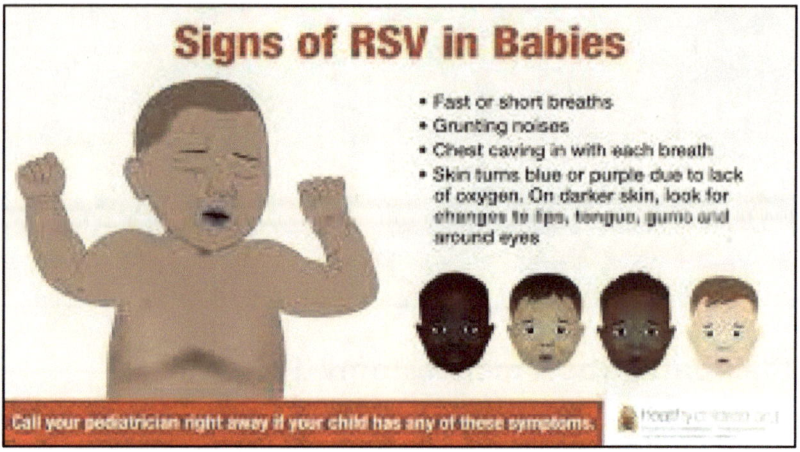

Suctioning Procedure:

Gather Supplies:

- Sterile suction catheter
- Suction machine with appropriate pressure (typically 80–120 mmHg for pediatrics)
- Saline to hydrate secretions (if needed)

Wash Hands and Wear Gloves:

Hand hygiene is critical for preventing infection.

Prepare Suction Machine:

- Check settings (appropriate suction pressure for the child's age and size).
- Ensure the suction canister and tubing are in place.

Suctioning Technique:

- Insert the catheter into the trach tube (don't force it).
- Suction while withdrawing the catheter—never leave the catheter in for more than 5-10 seconds.
- Use intermittent suctioning: apply suction as needed, but avoid prolonged suctioning to prevent trauma to the airway.
- Rinse the catheter with sterile saline between suction attempts if needed.

Post-Suction Care:

- Reassess the child's breathing, oxygen saturation, and comfort.
- Reposition the child if needed.
- Document the suctioning procedure, including the amount and type of secretions.

3. Changing the Tracheostomy Tube

Why Tube Changes Are Necessary:

Tracheostomy tubes need to be replaced periodically due to the buildup of secretions, tube wear, or in case of infection. Tube changes should be done per the physician's orders, but it's often done on a routine schedule (every 1–3 weeks).

Changing the Tracheostomy Tube Steps:

Prepare Supplies:

- New trach tube of the correct size and one size smaller
- Obturator
- Suctioning equipment
- Sterile saline and gauze
- Trach tube ties (if used)

Position the Child:

Position the child comfortably, with their head supported to keep the airway open.

Remove the Old Tube:

- Suction the child if needed to clear secretions.
- Loosen or remove the ties securing the old trach tube.
- Gently remove the old trach tube from the stoma.

Insert the New Tube:

- Insert the new trach tube with an obturator in place to guide it (don't remove the obturator until the tube is securely in position).
- Secure the new tube with fresh ties or Velcro straps.

- Check that the tube is positioned properly—there should be no resistance or signs of distress when the child breathes.

Post-Procedure Care:

- Suction if needed to clear any excess secretions after the tube is replaced.
- Reassess the child's oxygen saturation and respiratory rate.
- Document the procedure in detail: size of tube, any complications, and the child's response.

4. Managing Trach Emergencies

While rare, emergencies can occur with a trach tube. It's essential to stay calm, act quickly, and know how to manage common issues.

EMERGENCY SITUATION 1: Accidental Decannulation (Trach Tube Comes Out)

Stay Calm and Assess the Situation:

- Reposition the child's head and neck to keep the airway open.
- If the stoma is fresh (within a few days), you may need to reinsert the trach tube or use an ambu bag for resuscitation.
- If reinsertion is not possible, place a clean, sterile dressing over the stoma and call for emergency help immediately.

If the Child Can't Be Reintubated:

- Use the ambu bag to provide manual ventilation while waiting for emergency personnel.
- Prepare for emergency transport if needed.

EMERGENCY SITUATION 2: Blocked Trach Tube (Mucus or Other Obstruction)

Suction the Airway Immediately:

If the child is unable to breathe or is struggling, suction the tube thoroughly to remove any obstruction.

Reassess and Replace the Tube (if needed):

If suctioning doesn't clear the blockage, prepare to change the tube (with the new one that's already sized).

EMERGENCY SITUATION 3: Tube Displacement or Compromise (Signs of Infection or Damage)

Assess the Tube:

If the trach tube is compromised (e.g., cracked, leaking air), replace it immediately, using the spare tube you have on hand.

Monitor for Signs of Infection:

Fever, increased secretions, or swelling around the stoma may indicate an infection, which requires immediate attention and physician contact.

5. Routine Trach Care and Cleaning

Daily Care Routine:

- Clean the trach tube ties daily to prevent skin irritation.
- Inspect the stoma for signs of infection (redness, swelling, discharge).
- Clean the trach tube itself weekly, if not changed, by removing it and soaking it in saline or a sterile cleaning solution as recommended by the care team.

Tracheostomy position

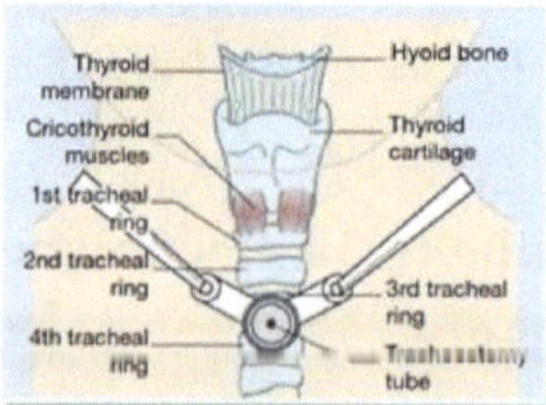

Tracheostomy tube

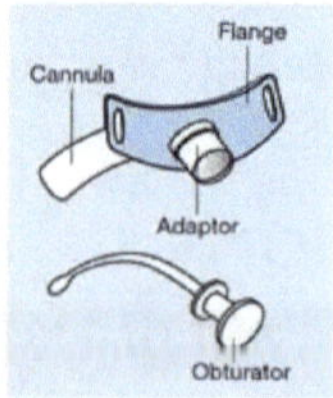

Suction technique

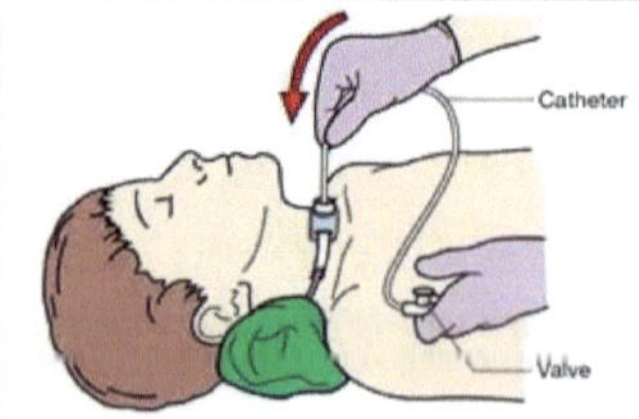

Equipment list for tape changes

Tape change equipment:

- Emergency box, oxygen and suction
- Gauze and saline
- 2 lengths of cotton/Velcro ties
- Scissors
- Rolled-up towel
- Blanket for swaddling
- Gloves and apron
- Child's comforter (e.g. dummy)

Tape change procedure

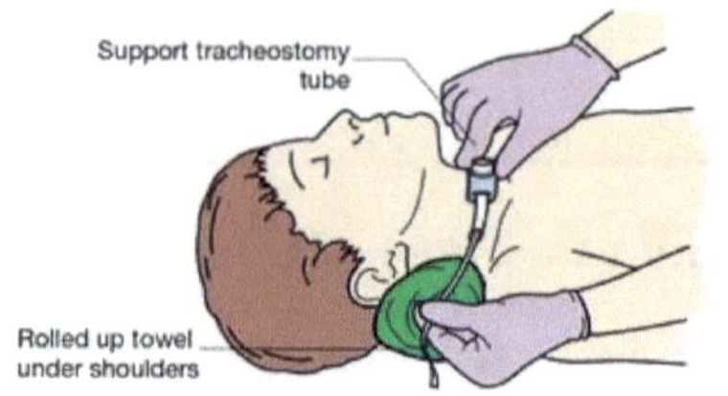

Checking tape tension

One finger should slip comfortably between the ties and the child's neck

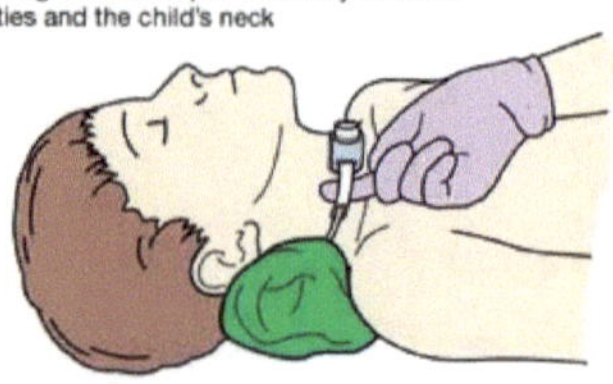

Equipment list for planned tube changes

Tube change equipment:

- Emergency box, oxygen and suction
- A tracheostomy tube same size and one size smaller
- 2 x syringes if child has cuffed tube
- Gauze and saline
- 2 lengths of cotton/Velcro ties
- Scissors
- Rolled-up towel
- Blanket for swaddling
- Gloves and apron
- Child's comforter (e.g. dummy)

Example of an emergency box

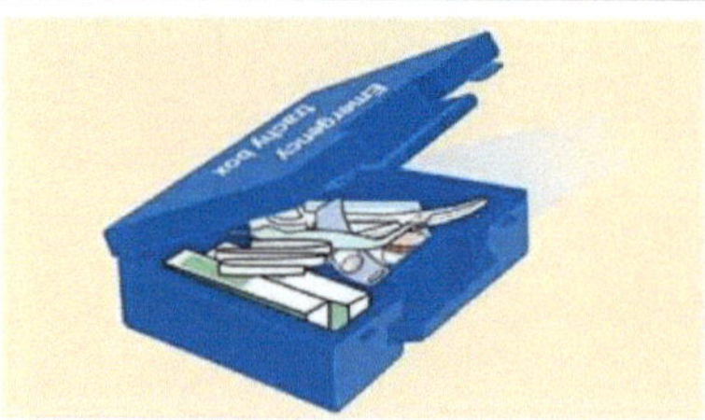

Contents of an emergency box

Emergency tracheostomy box contents:

- ✔ Same size tracheostomy + smaller size
- ✔ Tracheostomy tapes
- ✔ Disconnection wedge
- ✔ Scissors
- ✔ Lubricating jelly
- ✔ Syringes for cuffed tube
- ✔ Suction catheters

REMEMBER TO ALWAYS KNOW WHERE THE EMERGENCY BOX IS WHEN CARING FOR A CHILD WITH A TRACHEOSTOMY

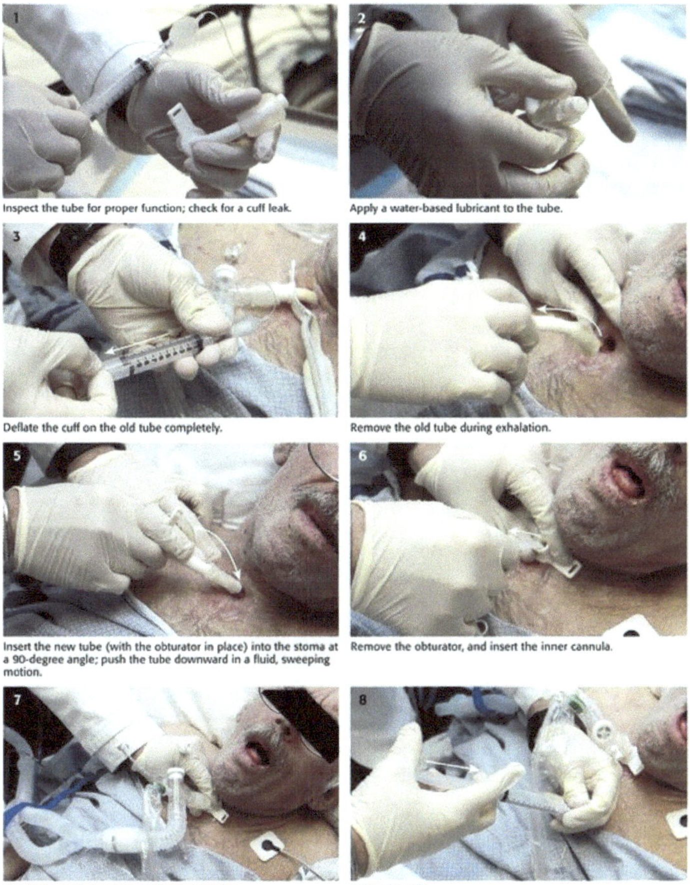

CHANGING A TRACHEOSTOMY TUBE

1 Inspect the tube for proper function; check for a cuff leak.

2 Apply a water-based lubricant to the tube.

3 Deflate the cuff on the old tube completely.

4 Remove the old tube during exhalation.

5 Insert the new tube (with the obturator in place) into the stoma at a 90-degree angle; push the tube downward in a fluid, sweeping motion.

6 Remove the obturator, and insert the inner cannula.

7 Attach the ventilator to the tracheostomy tube.

8 Inflate the cuff.

6. Trach Care Tips for Success

- ***Stay prepared:*** Always have spare trach tubes (in the correct size) and an obturator ready.
- ***Build rapport with the family:*** Make sure the family knows how to help with emergency situations and tube changes if they are able.
- ***Stay alert:*** The airway can change quickly—never wait too long before suctioning or reassessing if the child's breathing seems off.
- ***Communicate with the rest of the care team:*** Regularly update the medical team on the child's airway health, especially after any issues arise.

CHAPTER 7
G-Tube Care

A Detailed Guide to G-Tube Management, Feeding, and Complications

Gastrostomy tubes (G-tubes) are commonly used in pediatric homecare to provide long-term feeding support when oral feeding is not possible or safe. G-tube care requires routine attention to prevent complications and ensure the child receives the correct nutrition. This chapter covers everything you need to know about G-tube care, from insertion to troubleshooting potential problems.

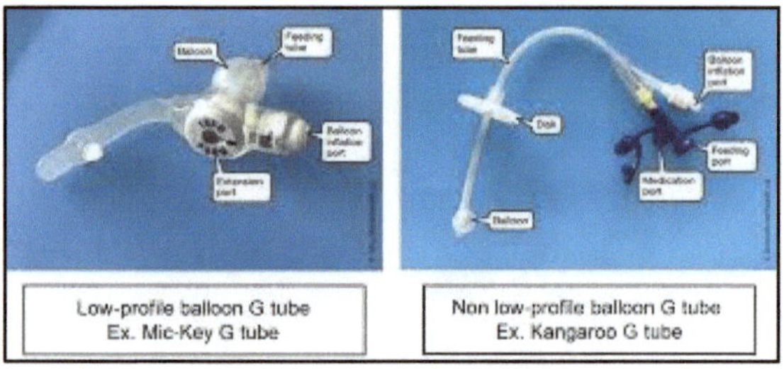

Low-profile balloon G tube
Ex. Mic-Key G tube

Non low-profile balloon G tube
Ex. Kangaroo G tube

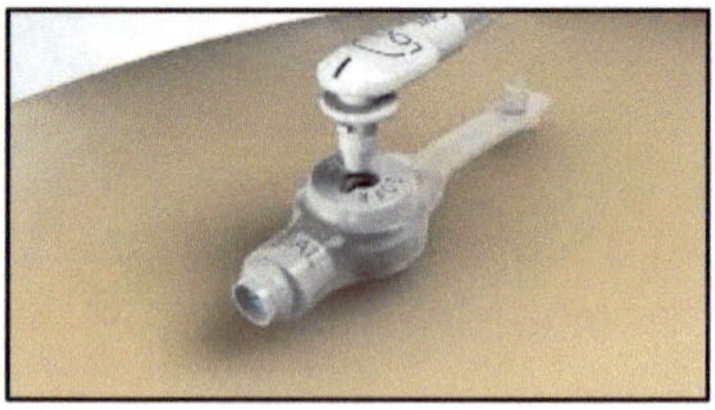

1. Understanding G-Tubes: Purpose and Placement

What Is a G-Tube?

A G-tube is a surgically placed feeding tube that provides direct access to the stomach through the abdominal wall. It's used in cases where a child is unable to eat or drink orally due to medical conditions like neurological disorders, congenital abnormalities, or chronic conditions.

Types of G-Tubes:

- ***PEG (Percutaneous Endoscopic Gastrostomy):*** Inserted via an endoscopic procedure, commonly used for long-term feeding.

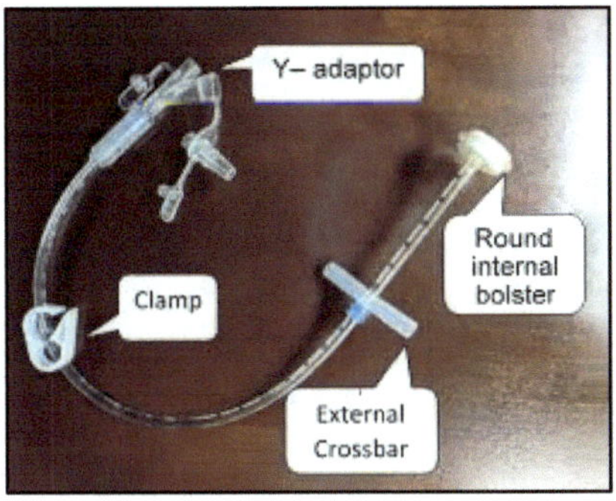

- ***Low-profile G-Tube (Button):*** A small, discreet device often preferred for older children or those who have more mobility.

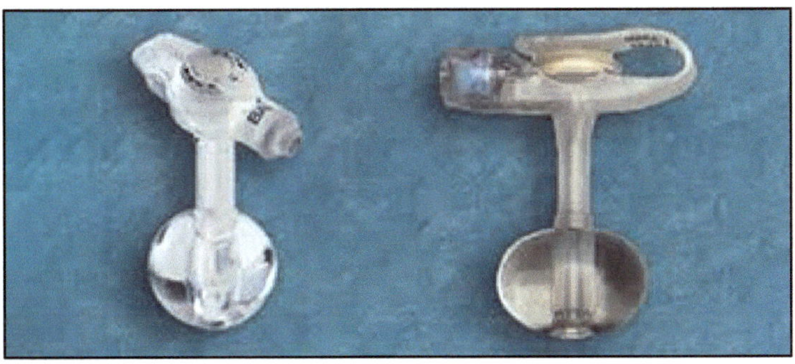

- ***G-J Tube (Gastric-Jejunal):*** A tube that goes from the stomach into the jejunum, often used for children who have severe reflux or aspiration risks.

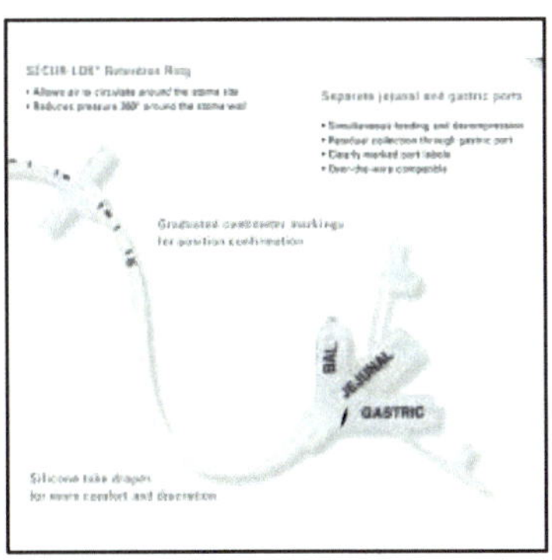

2. Inserting and Maintaining a G-Tube

Post-Insertion Care:

The first few weeks after G-tube placement are crucial, as the stoma (hole in the abdomen) must heal properly to prevent infection and leakage. This period is critical for ensuring that both the tube and the site are kept clean and secure.

Insertion Site Care:

- ***Inspect the G-tube site:*** Look for signs of infection such as redness, swelling, or drainage.
- ***Keep the site clean:*** Clean around the stoma with warm water and mild soap, especially before and after feedings. Avoid using alcohol-based cleansers unless directed by a physician.
- ***Secure the Tube:*** Make sure the tube is not pulling or tugging on the skin, as this can lead to irritation or premature dislodgement.

Routine Tube Maintenance:

- Change the dressing around the G-tube as needed, generally every 1-3 days, or if it becomes wet or soiled.
- Rotate the G-tube gently (a quarter turn) during cleaning to prevent skin adherence to the tube.
- Use sterile or distilled water to flush the tube before and after feedings or medication administration to prevent clogging.

3. Feeding via G-Tube

Types of Feedings:

- ***Bolus Feeding:*** Larger volumes of formula or food are given at set intervals (e.g., every 4-6 hours). This method mimics normal eating patterns and is often preferred for children who can tolerate larger feedings.

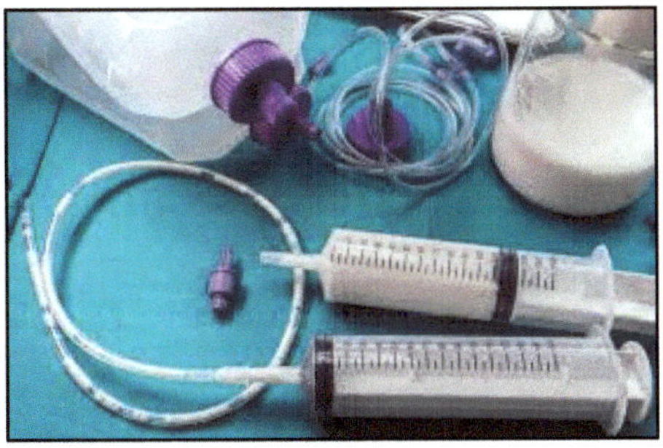

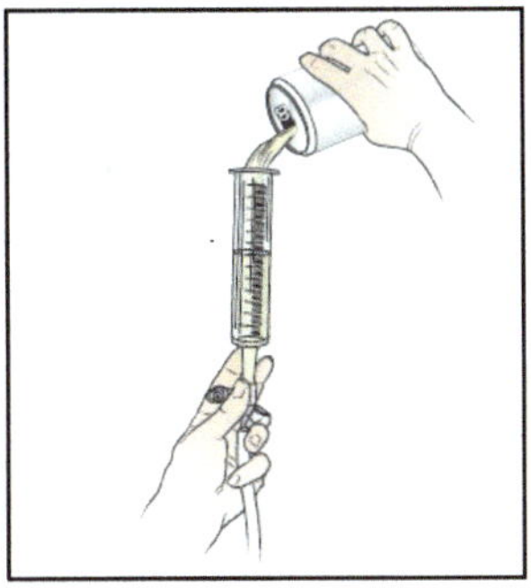

- ***Continuous Feeding:*** Formula is delivered slowly over a period of time, typically 12-24 hours. This is often used for children who have feeding intolerance or slower gastric emptying.

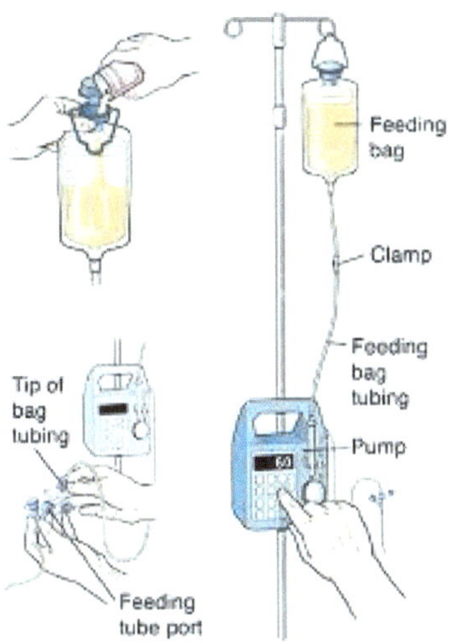

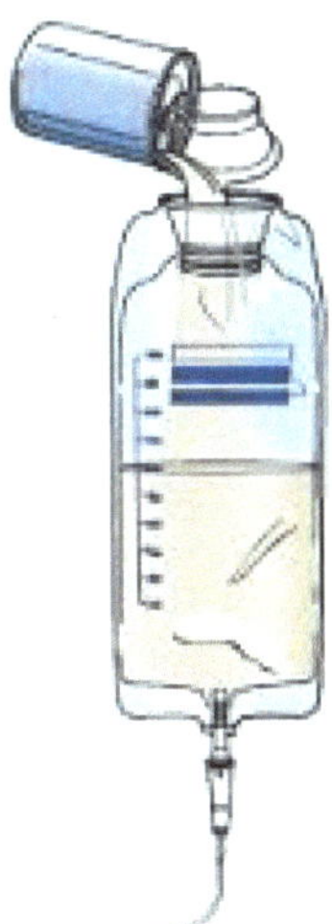

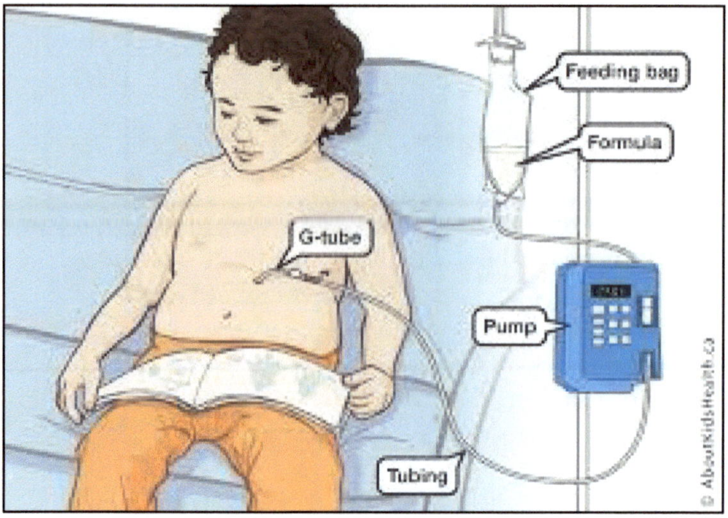

- ***Supplemental Feedings:*** In some cases, the G-tube is used to provide extra calories or hydration between oral feedings.

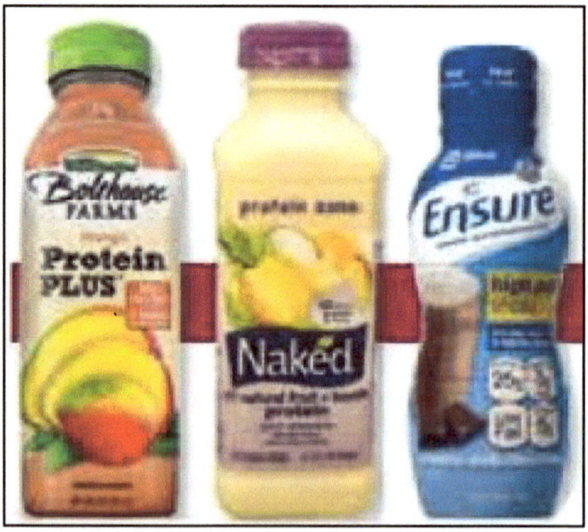

Steps for Administering a Bolus Feeding:

Prepare the Feeding Solution:

- Verify the formula and amount prescribed.
- Make sure the formula is at room temperature—cold or warm formula can cause discomfort.
- Check that the feeding syringe or bag is clean and ready to use.

Flush the Tube:

Flush the tube with sterile water or saline to ensure patency before administering the feeding.

Administer the Feeding:

- Attach the syringe to the G-tube port, and slowly push the formula in. Ensure the formula is delivered at a slow and steady pace to prevent nausea or discomfort.
- If using a feeding bag, hang it above the child's stomach and allow the formula to flow at a consistent rate.
- Keep the child in an upright position during and after the feeding to prevent reflux and aspiration.

Post-Feeding Care:

- Flush the tube again with sterile water to clear any remaining formula and prevent clogging.
- Check the child for any signs of discomfort, bloating, or gagging.
- Clean the feeding equipment after each use and store it properly.

4. G-Tube Complications and Troubleshooting

While G-tubes are generally safe, there are potential complications that you must be prepared to handle.

Complication 1: Tube Clogging

Clogging can happen if food or medication is not properly flushed through the tube.

How to Prevent:

- Always flush the tube before and after feedings or medications.
- Use warm water to dissolve any blockage before attempting to clear it.

How to Clear:

- Try gently flushing with warm water.
- If the blockage doesn't clear, use a syringe with a little force to clear the tube.

- If the tube remains clogged, contact the physician for advice or a replacement tube.

Complication 2: Skin Irritation or Infection

This can occur around the stoma, leading to discomfort or infection.

Prevention:

- Keep the area clean and dry.
- Use a gentle, non-alcoholic cleanser to clean around the site.
- Avoid tight clothing or straps that might irritate the area.

Treatment:

- If redness or discharge is noted, apply an antibiotic ointment as prescribed.
- If the area becomes increasingly painful, swollen, or if there's pus, notify the physician immediately.

Complication 3: Tube Dislodgement

Sometimes, the G-tube can become loose or dislodged, which can be an emergency if the stoma has not fully healed.

Immediate Action:

- If the tube becomes dislodged and the stoma is not fully healed, cover the area with a clean, sterile dressing and seek immediate medical attention.
- For a dislodged but healed tube, you may need to replace the tube yourself, if trained, or contact emergency services.

5. G-Tube Emergency Procedures

Emergency 1: Tube Dislodgement

If the tube becomes dislodged, immediately assess if the stoma is healed. If it's newly placed, don't attempt reinsertion. Instead, cover the hole with a clean dressing and call for emergency help.

Emergency 2: Aspirating Feeding (Risk of Aspiration)

Monitor the child closely during and after feedings for signs of aspiration, such as coughing, choking, or a change in respiratory effort. Always keep the child in an upright position for 30 minutes after feeding.

6. Routine G-Tube Care: Tips for Success

- ***Consistency is Key:*** Regular cleaning and flushing are essential to preventing blockages and infections.
- ***Monitor for Complications:*** Keep a close eye on the skin around the tube and any signs of irritation or infection.
- ***Know Your Emergency Protocols:*** Have a plan for dislodgement, aspiration, and other emergencies. Always have a spare tube on hand.
- ***Educate the Family:*** Teach parents or caregivers the basics of tube care, feeding, and troubleshooting to ensure they are confident in managing the G-tube between nursing visits.

CHAPTER 8
Medication Management and Administration

A Step-by-Step Guide to Safe Medication Administration in Pediatric Homecare

Administering medications in a homecare setting can be complex, especially when the child has a G-tube or tracheostomy. It's crucial to follow prescribed schedules, monitor for side effects, and ensure that each medication is given through the correct route. This chapter will guide you through the processes for administering medications via G-tube, oral route, or injections, as well as tips for safety and troubleshooting.

1. Types of Medications in Pediatric Homecare

In pediatric homecare, a variety of medications may be administered to manage the child's condition, including:

- ***Oral Medications:*** Pills, tablets, liquids, or dissolving medications
- ***Tube-Administered Medications:*** G-tube, J-tube, or NG-tube
- ***Injectable Medications:*** Subcutaneous, intramuscular, or intravenous
- ***Topical Medications:*** Creams, ointments, or patches
- ***Inhaled Medications:*** Nebulized treatments or inhalers, often used for respiratory conditions

2. General Medication Safety Guidelines

1. Medication Verification:

- Always verify the medication before administration:
- The child's name and date of birth
- The medication name, dosage, route, and time
- The expiration date and the drug label for instructions

2. Hand Hygiene:

Always wash your hands before handling medications to reduce the risk of contamination. Wear gloves if necessary, especially when administering via the G-tube.

3. Correct Dosage and Route:

Administer medications according to the doctor's orders. Ensure that the correct dosage is given, and that the route (oral, G-tube, etc.) is followed. If you have any doubts about dosage or route, consult the prescribing physician or pharmacist.

4. Medication Storage:

Store medications in a cool, dry place, as instructed. Keep them out of reach of children and pets.

3. Oral Medication Administration

Administering Oral Medications:

For children who are able to swallow, oral medications are straightforward. However, for those with a G-tube or other feeding tubes, oral medications must be crushed or liquidized.

Steps for Oral Medication Administration:

Verify Medication:

- Check the medication's label, dosage, and timing.
- Ensure the child is in an appropriate position for swallowing, such as sitting up to prevent aspiration.

Give the Medication:

- If the child can swallow, offer the medication with a drink of water or juice.
- For those who can't swallow pills, crush tablets or open capsules (if safe) and mix with a small amount of liquid or food, as instructed by the physician or pharmacist.

Monitor for Side Effects:

Watch for any signs of discomfort, allergic reactions, or changes in the child's behavior. Report any adverse effects to the physician.

4. Medication Administration via G-Tube

Administering Medication via G-Tube:

When giving medication via a G-tube, special care is needed to prevent clogging, ensure proper absorption, and avoid aspiration. Medication must be in the correct form (liquid or crushed tablets mixed with water).

Steps for G-Tube Medication Administration:

Prepare the Medication:

- If giving liquid medication, ensure it is at room temperature and ready to administer.
- If the medication is in pill form, crush the tablet (only if allowed by the prescribing doctor) and mix with a small amount of water.
- For capsules, check if they can be opened. If so, mix the contents with water or juice.

Check Tube Patency:

Always flush the G-tube with 15-30 mL of sterile water or saline before and after administering medication. This clears the tube of any residual formula or food and ensures the medication will be absorbed.

Administer the Medication:

Pour the medication into the syringe and slowly push it into the G-tube. Allow it to flow at a controlled pace to avoid reflux or discomfort.

Post-Medication Care:

- After administering the medication, flush the tube again with sterile water or saline to clear any remaining medication.
- Document the medication, time, and any issues that may have occurred (e.g., resistance, discomfort).

5. Injectable Medications

Injectable medications, such as insulin, growth hormones, or emergency medications, may be required in some cases. It's important to follow proper injection techniques to minimize pain, risk of infection, and ensure the medication is delivered effectively.

Steps for Administering Injectable Medications:

Prepare the Medication:

- Check the expiration date, type of medication, and route (subcutaneous, intramuscular, etc.).
- Draw up the correct amount of medication into the syringe, ensuring no air bubbles are present.

Select the Injection Site:

- Choose an appropriate injection site (e.g., fatty tissue for subcutaneous injections or muscle for intramuscular).
- Rotate injection sites to avoid tissue damage or irritation.

Administer the Injection:

- Clean the injection site with an alcohol wipe.
- Insert the needle at the correct angle (typically 45-90 degrees, depending on the type of injection).
- Inject the medication slowly and steadily.

Post-Injection Care:

- Apply gentle pressure to the site with a clean gauze to prevent bleeding.
- Dispose of the needle and syringe in a proper sharps container.

6. Managing Medication Schedules

Create a Medication Log:

- Maintain a daily log of all medications given, including time, dosage, route, and any reactions.
- Ensure that the log is easily accessible to family members or caregivers to follow the schedule when the nurse is not present.

Set Reminders:

- Set alarms or use medication reminder apps to ensure medications are administered on time.
- Some families may also find it helpful to have a medication management sheet for easy tracking.

DRUG	TYPE	TRADE NAMES	ADMINISTRATION
Short Acting			
albuterol	$Beta_2$	Proventil, Ventolin	PO, inhalation
ephedrine	Alpha/beta	None (various generic)	IM, IV, subcut
epinephrine	Alpha/beta	Adrenalin	Subcut, IM
metaproterenol	$Beta_1/beta_2$	Alupent	PO, inhalation
levalbuterol	$Beta_2$	Xopenex	Inhalation
metaproterenol	$Beta_1/beta_2$	Alupent, Metaprel	PO, inhalation
pirbuterol	$Beta_2$	Maxair	Inhalation
terbutaline	$Beta_2$	Brethine	PO, subcut, inhalation
Long Acting			
salmeterol	$Beta_2$	Serevent, Serevent Diskus	Inhalation
formoterol	$Beta_2$	Foradil, Perforomist	Inhalation
arformoterol	$Beta_2$	Brovana	Inhalation

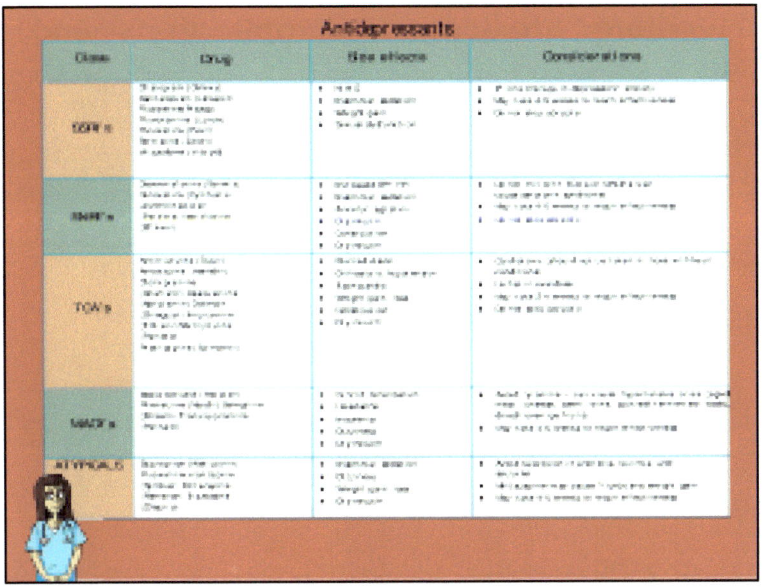
Antidepressants
Class
Drug
Side effects
Considerations
SSRI's
SNRI's
TCA's
MAOI's
ATYPICALS

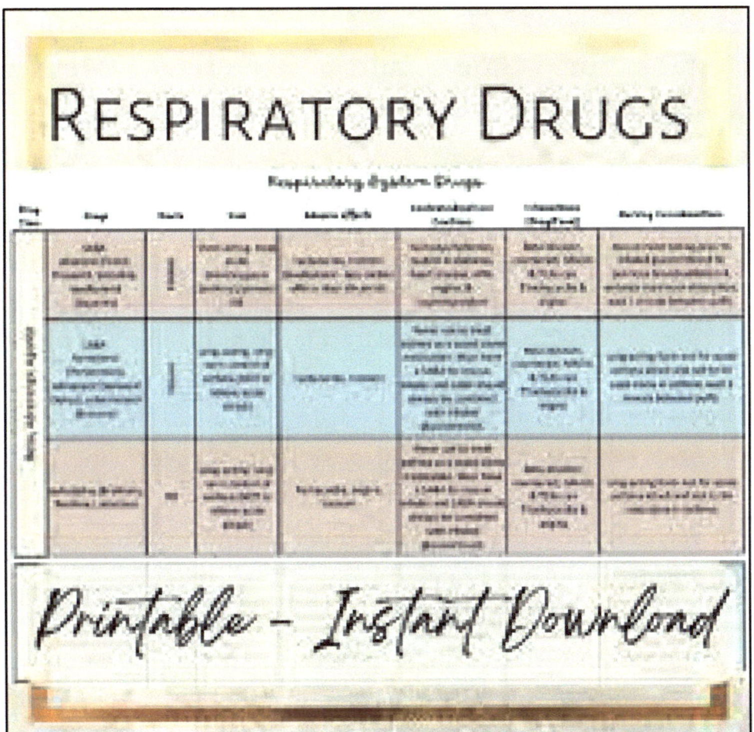
RESPIRATORY DRUGS
Respiratory System Drugs
Printable - Instant Download

7. Handling Medication Complications and Side Effects

Allergic Reactions:

Signs of an allergic reaction include swelling, rash, difficulty breathing, or hives. If any of these symptoms occur, stop administering the medication and seek medical help immediately.

Medication Interactions:

Some medications may interact with others, leading to decreased effectiveness or side effects. Always consult the prescribing physician or pharmacist before adding new medications or supplements.

Vomiting or Regurgitation After Medication:

If the child vomits immediately after taking oral or G-tube medication, check with the physician to see if the dose should be repeated.

8. Tips for Safe and Effective Medication Administration

- ***Use Correct Measuring Tools:*** Always use a syringe or medicine cup with proper measurements to ensure the correct dosage.
- ***Double-Check Dosages:*** If you are administering medications with varying dosages, always verify the correct amount.
- ***Avoid Mixing Medications:*** Don't mix different medications together in the same syringe unless specifically instructed by a healthcare provider.
- ***Monitor the Child's Response:*** Always check the child after administration for signs of adverse reactions.
- ***Stop the feed.*** Flush the tube with an appropriate amount of water. Ensure the tube is clean.
- ***Administer one medication at a time.*** Prepare all medicines and dilutions just before administration.
- ***Draw up liquid formulations using a syringe for accurate dosing.*** Crush tablets or open capsules and disperse in a set amount of water according to pharmacist's instructions, and measure out the dose using a syringe.

- ***Attach the syringe to the tube and apply gentle pressure***
- ***Flush well with water between medications.*** Flush well after all the medications are administered. Ensure the tube is clean.

CHAPTER 9
Personal Care and Hygiene

A Comprehensive Guide to Daily Hygiene, Skin Care, and Comfort for Pediatric Homecare Patients

Personal care and hygiene are vital aspects of maintaining overall health and comfort for children receiving homecare, particularly those with complex medical needs like tracheostomies and G-tubes. Proper hygiene routines help prevent infections, promote skin integrity, and support emotional well-being. This chapter will provide a step-by-step guide for managing the personal care of pediatric patients, including bathing, skin care, and other hygiene practices.

1. Daily Hygiene Care: Bathing and Skin Care

Children in homecare may have limited mobility or require specific adaptations during personal care routines. Bathing, skin care, and grooming must be approached with care to avoid irritation, discomfort, or injury, especially for children with medical devices like a tracheostomy or feeding tube.

Bathing and Showering:

Frequency:

Bathing frequency depends on the child's needs and condition. Generally, a full bath or shower is recommended 2-3 times a week, but more frequent cleaning may be needed for children with incontinence, sweating, or other specific needs.

Preparation:

- Ensure that the bathroom is warm, comfortable, and free of any items that could pose a safety risk.
- Have all necessary bathing supplies within reach (e.g., soap, washcloths, towels, clean clothes).
- Ensure that any medical equipment, such as the tracheostomy tube, is properly covered to avoid exposure to water (use waterproof dressings or covers).

Steps for Bathing:

Safety First:

If the child has a trach tube, ensure that the dressing is secure and that the airway is protected from water exposure. You may want to cover the trach with a waterproof bandage or use a shower shield for extra protection.

Gentle Cleansing:

- Use mild, non-irritating soap and warm water to cleanse the child's body.
- Avoid harsh soaps or products that could dry or irritate the skin, especially around the tracheostomy site or G-tube stoma.

Drying and Moisturizing:

- Pat the child's skin dry with a clean towel.
- Apply a gentle, fragrance-free moisturizer to prevent dryness or irritation, particularly around the G-tube and trach site, where skin can become more sensitive.

Hair Care:

- If the child has hair, gently wash and rinse with baby shampoo or a mild shampoo to avoid scalp irritation.
- Dry and comb hair carefully to prevent tangles and discomfort.

2. Tracheostomy and G-Tube Site Care

Maintaining cleanliness and preventing infection at the tracheostomy and G-tube insertion sites is critical. Both areas require careful daily inspection and hygiene routines to prevent complications like infection, irritation, or skin breakdown.

Tracheostomy Site Care:

Inspect for Infection:

- Check the skin around the stoma for signs of infection (redness, swelling, discharge).
- If there is any indication of infection, report it to the physician.

Clean the Stoma Area:

- Use warm water and mild soap to clean the skin around the tracheostomy site.
- Avoid using alcohol-based products, as they can cause dryness or irritation.

Dry Thoroughly:

- Pat the stoma area dry with a clean towel.
- Apply a thin layer of protective ointment or barrier cream around the stoma if advised by the physician.

Trach Tube and Dressing Change:

- Change the tracheostomy dressing regularly to keep the area clean and dry.
- Always use sterile or clean technique when handling the trach tube to reduce the risk of infection.

G-Tube Site Care:

Inspect for Signs of Infection:

Check the G-tube stoma site daily for redness, discharge, or signs of infection. If there are any concerns, notify the physician.

Clean the Insertion Site:

- Gently clean around the stoma with warm water and mild soap.
- Rotate the G-tube gently (a quarter turn) during cleaning to prevent skin irritation and to avoid the tube adhering to the skin.

Skin Protection:

Apply a clean dressing or gauze around the G-tube site to absorb moisture and prevent friction. Change this dressing as needed.

Tube Maintenance:

- Keep the tube securely in place to avoid pulling on the stoma or causing discomfort.
- Flush the tube regularly with sterile water to ensure it remains patent.

3. Oral Care and Hygiene

Proper oral hygiene is especially important for children with tracheostomies or feeding tubes, as poor oral health can lead to respiratory infections or other complications. If the child has a trach, regular oral care is critical to prevent aspiration pneumonia or infection.

Steps for Oral Care:

Brush Teeth Daily:

Use a soft toothbrush and non-alcoholic toothpaste. Brush the child's teeth at least twice a day to remove plaque and prevent cavities.

Clean the Mouth (for Non-Oral Feeders):

Even if the child cannot eat orally, use a soft toothbrush or mouth swab to clean the mouth, gums, and tongue. This helps prevent infections and keeps the mouth fresh.

Mouth Rinses:

If recommended by the physician, use a saline solution or alcohol-free mouthwash to rinse the mouth and clear away bacteria.

Hydrate the Mouth:

For children who are not drinking fluids orally, provide moisture with a saline spray or by swabbing the mouth with a damp cloth to prevent dryness and irritation.

4. Nail Care and Grooming

Nail care is an important part of hygiene and personal care. Long or sharp nails can cause injury to the child or lead to skin infections.

Steps for Nail Care:

Check for Length:

- Regularly trim the child's nails to prevent scratches or potential injury.
- Always use child-safe nail clippers or scissors.

Soften Nails Before Cutting:

If the nails are hard, consider soaking them in warm water to soften them before cutting.

Clean Under Nails:

After trimming, gently clean under the nails using a soft nail brush or washcloth to remove any debris.

5. Skin Care and Moisturizing

Children with feeding tubes or tracheostomies are at increased risk for skin breakdown or irritation, particularly around the insertion sites. Keeping the skin hydrated and free from friction is key to preventing complications.

Skin Care Tips:

Moisturize Daily:

Apply a gentle, fragrance-free moisturizer to the child's skin, especially in areas prone to dryness (e.g., around the trach site or G-tube stoma).

Prevent Friction:

Use soft fabrics and avoid tight clothing that can rub against the skin and cause irritation.

Make sure medical equipment, such as trach ties or feeding tube straps, is not too tight and doesn't cause chafing.

Check for Pressure Sores:

Regularly inspect areas where the child may experience pressure (e.g., back, ears, or under straps). Use soft padding if needed to prevent skin breakdown.

6. Preventing Infection and Promoting Comfort

Maintaining good hygiene and skin care routines helps to prevent infections and keeps the child comfortable. Always report any signs of infection, discomfort, or abnormal changes in skin condition to the healthcare team.

CHAPTER 10
Emergency Procedures and Crisis Management

A Comprehensive Guide to Managing Emergencies in Pediatric Homecare

Caring for a pediatric patient with medical complexities such as a tracheostomy, G-tube, or other medical needs requires preparedness for emergencies. While many situations can be managed calmly and effectively with the right knowledge, it's essential to know how to respond quickly and confidently during a crisis. This chapter covers the most common emergencies you may encounter in pediatric home nursing, including respiratory distress, tube dislodgement, aspiration, and other urgent situations.

1. Recognizing Respiratory Distress and Emergencies

For children with a tracheostomy or other respiratory conditions, monitoring breathing is critical. Respiratory distress can develop quickly and may lead to life-threatening situations if not addressed promptly.

Signs of Respiratory Distress:

- ***Increased work of breathing:*** Look for signs of labored or rapid breathing, such as flaring nostrils, chest retractions (the skin around the ribs pulling in), or grunting.
- ***Changes in skin color:*** Cyanosis (a bluish color around the lips, face, or extremities) or pallor (paleness) indicate insufficient oxygen levels.
- ***Noisy breathing or wheezing:*** Any change in the sound of the child's breathing, such as wheezing, stridor, or gurgling, should be immediately addressed.
- ***Restlessness or anxiety:*** The child may appear distressed or agitated if they are struggling to breathe.

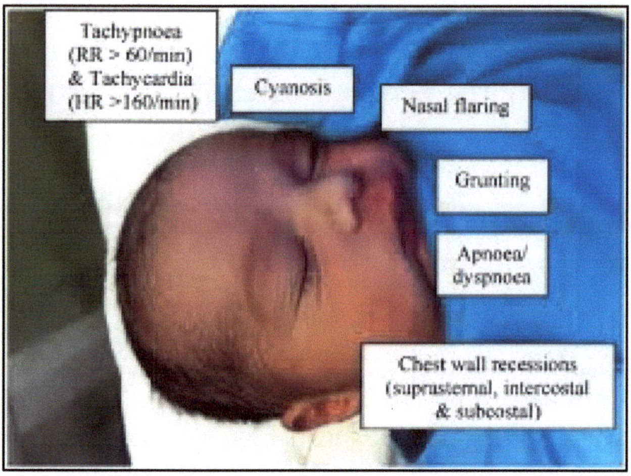

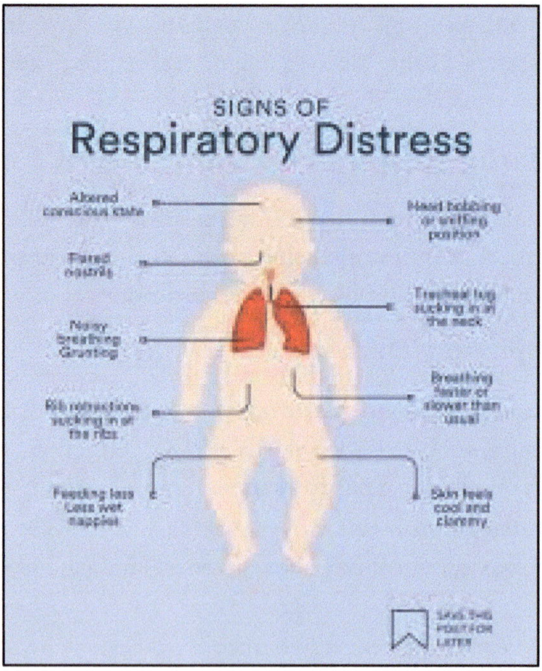

Immediate Action for Respiratory Distress:

Check the Airway:

- Ensure the tracheostomy tube is patent (open). If the tube is blocked, clear it immediately by suctioning or removing the obstruction.

- If there is a mucous plug in the trach, perform suctioning (if trained) or use saline to loosen the mucus.
- If the trach tube is dislodged, follow the procedure for re-insertion, or if unable to do so, call emergency services immediately.

Administer Oxygen (if prescribed):

- If the child has a prescribed oxygen regimen, ensure it is being delivered at the correct flow rate.
- Use supplemental oxygen via nasal cannula, oxygen mask, or a ventilator if the child's condition warrants it.

Monitor Vital Signs:

Keep an eye on the child's pulse, oxygen saturation (SpO2), and heart rate. A significant decrease in oxygen saturation is a critical sign of respiratory compromise.

Contact Emergency Services:

If the child's breathing does not improve with basic interventions or if the situation becomes life-threatening, contact emergency medical services (EMS) immediately.

2. Handling Tube Dislodgement (Tracheostomy or G-Tube)

Tube dislodgement can be a medical emergency, particularly if the stoma has not fully healed. Timely action can prevent complications such as airway obstruction or difficulty feeding.

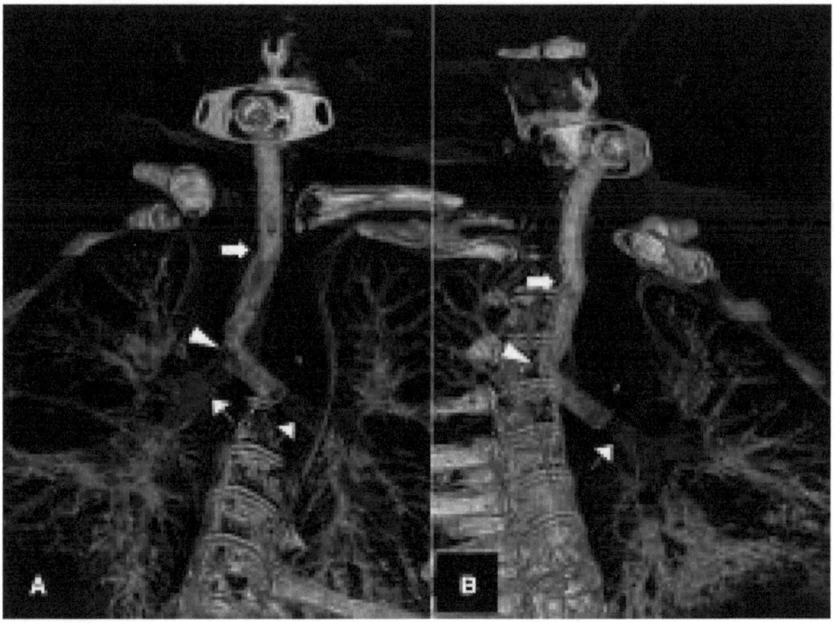

Tracheostomy Tube Dislodgement:

For a Newly Inserted Tube:

If the trach tube is newly placed (within the first 1-2 weeks), cover the stoma with a clean, sterile dressing. Do not attempt to replace the tube; immediately call for emergency medical help.

For an Older, Healed Stoma:

- If the tube becomes dislodged and the stoma has healed, you may be able to reinsert the tube yourself if you've been trained.
- Always have a spare tracheostomy tube of the correct size and type available in case of emergency.
- If reinsertion is unsuccessful or you're unsure, seek emergency medical assistance immediately.

G-Tube Dislodgement:

For a Newly Inserted G-Tube:

If the G-tube becomes dislodged and the stoma is not healed, cover the site with a sterile dressing. Contact medical personnel for advice on how to proceed.

For an Established G-Tube:

- If the G-tube is dislodged and the site is healed, a replacement tube may be inserted, following the medical provider's instructions.
- If reinsertion is not possible, contact emergency services immediately.

3. Managing Aspiration and Choking

Aspiration occurs when food, liquid, or secretions enter the airway and can lead to aspiration pneumonia. Choking is a direct airway obstruction that can be life-threatening.

Signs of Aspiration:

- ***Coughing or gagging:*** The child may cough or gag during or after feeding.
- ***Changes in respiratory status:*** Difficulty breathing, wheezing, or sudden shortness of breath following a feeding can be a sign of aspiration.
- ***Fever or signs of pneumonia:*** Fever or difficulty breathing hours or days after a feeding episode can indicate aspiration pneumonia.

Immediate Action for Aspiration:

Clear the Airway:

- If the child is coughing or struggling to breathe, encourage them to cough to expel the material from the airway.
- For a child who cannot cough effectively, perform the Heimlich maneuver if trained and appropriate.
- Suctioning may be necessary if the airway is obstructed with secretions or food.

Administer Oxygen (if prescribed):

Provide supplemental oxygen if the child's oxygen levels drop.

Monitor for Complications:

Watch for signs of aspiration pneumonia, including persistent cough, fever, or difficulty breathing after an aspiration episode.

Seek Medical Attention:

If the child shows signs of aspiration, contact the physician or emergency services to evaluate for potential respiratory infections.

4. Seizures and Neurological Emergencies

Seizures can occur in children with neurological disorders or other conditions. Immediate intervention is necessary to ensure safety and prevent injury.

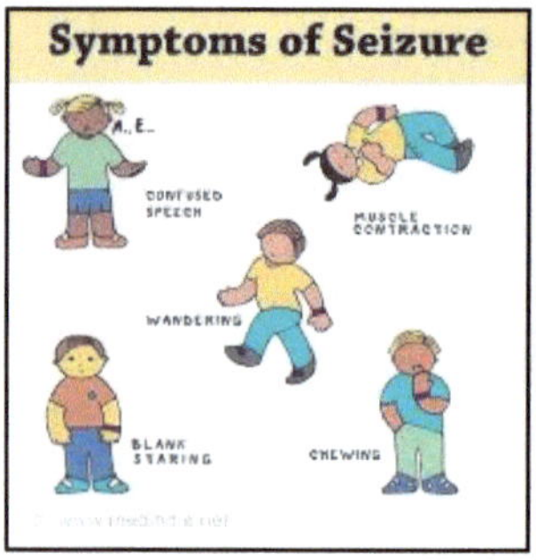

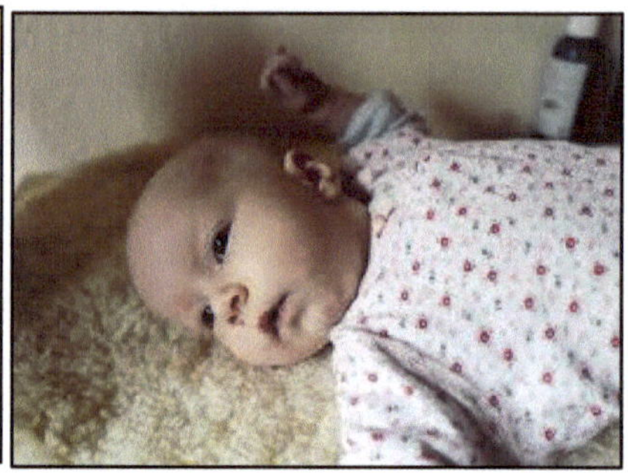

Signs of a Seizure:

- ***Tonic-Clonic Seizures:*** Stiffening of the body, followed by rhythmic jerking movements.
- ***Absence Seizures:*** Brief periods of unresponsiveness, staring, or blinking.

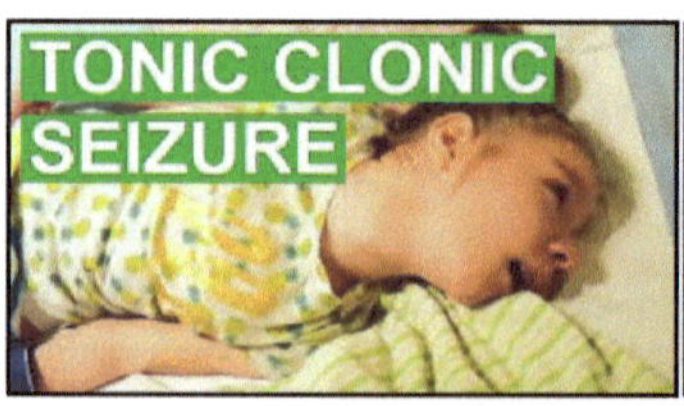

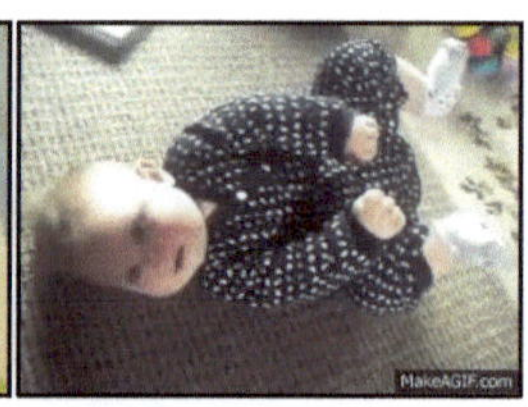

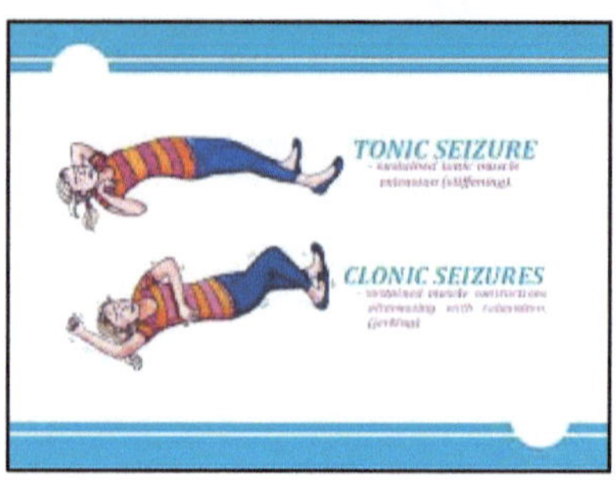

- ***Focal Seizures:*** Abnormal movements or sensations in one part of the body, such as twitching in a limb.

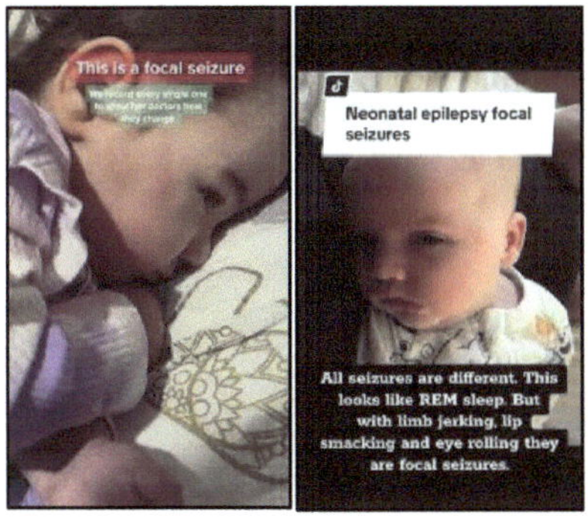

Immediate Action During a Seizure:

Ensure Safety:

- Keep the child safe by clearing the area of sharp objects or obstacles that could cause injury.
- Gently position the child on their side if possible to prevent choking or aspiration.

Time of the Seizure:

- Note the duration of the seizure. If it lasts longer than 5 minutes, call emergency services immediately.
- If the child has multiple seizures in a row without regaining consciousness, seek immediate medical attention.

Administer Rescue Medications (if prescribed):

If the child has a seizure management plan and rescue medications (e.g., diazepam or lorazepam), administer as instructed by the healthcare provider.

Post-Seizure Care:

- After the seizure, monitor the child for confusion, lethargy, or difficulty breathing.
- If necessary, provide comfort and reassurance as the child recovers.

5. Other Urgent Situations

Fever and Infection:

- ***Signs of Infection:*** Look for fever, increased heart rate, fatigue, irritability, and signs of local infection (redness, swelling, discharge at the G tube or tracheostomy site).
- ***Immediate Action:*** Administer fever-reducing medications as prescribed, provide fluids, and monitor vital signs. Contact the healthcare provider if the fever persists or if the child shows signs of dehydration or distress.

Bleeding:

- ***Minor Bleeding (e.g., from a G-tube or tracheostomy site):*** Apply gentle pressure with a sterile dressing to control bleeding.
- ***Severe Bleeding:*** If the bleeding does not stop with pressure or if the child is showing signs of significant blood loss, call for emergency medical help immediately.

6. When to Call Emergency Services

In any of the following cases, call emergency services immediately:

- Respiratory distress that does not improve with intervention
- Tube dislodgement that cannot be corrected
- Severe aspiration or choking episodes
- Seizures that last longer than 5 minutes or multiple seizures in a row
- Severe bleeding or signs of shock
- Fever with signs of infection that do not improve with medication

7. Preparing for Emergencies

Create an Emergency Kit:

Ensure you have essential supplies on hand, including spare tubes (trach and G-tube), suction equipment, rescue medications, and emergency contact information.

Know the Emergency Protocols:

Familiarize yourself with the family's care plan and emergency protocols. Ensure all caregivers are trained on what to do in an emergency.

Keep Emergency Contacts Accessible:

Have contact numbers for the child's healthcare team, local emergency services, and poison control readily available.

CHAPTER 11
Transitioning to Adult Care and Long-Term Planning

Preparing for the Future: Transitioning Pediatric Homecare to Adult Care

As children with complex medical needs grow older, the time will come to transition from pediatric to adult healthcare services. This process can be both challenging and empowering, requiring careful planning, communication, and support for the family and child. This chapter provides guidance on how to navigate the transition smoothly, ensuring that the child's medical needs continue to be met while also preparing them for greater independence and self-care.

1. Understanding the Transition to Adult Care

The transition from pediatric to adult care involves more than just switching doctors or clinics. It requires careful consideration of the child's medical, emotional, and social needs, as well as the involvement of the entire care team. Children who have been receiving homecare, including specialized treatments like tracheostomy care or G-tube management, will face new challenges as they age into adulthood.

Key Considerations:

Continuity of Care:

Ensure that the child's medical needs will continue to be addressed appropriately as they move to adult care. The adult healthcare system may operate differently than pediatric services, and it's essential to find providers who are experienced in managing the child's specific condition.

Medical Complexity:

Many young adults with chronic conditions require specialized care that is different from what they received as children. Adult physicians may need additional training to handle complex pediatric conditions.

Psychosocial Development:

As the child matures, their emotional and social needs will also evolve. Preparing the child for adult care requires addressing their growing sense of independence, self-esteem, and coping strategies.

2. Key Steps in Preparing for the Transition

Planning for the transition should begin early, ideally before the child turns 18. The goal is to prepare the child, family, and care team for the changes that will occur.

Start Early:

Discuss the Transition Process:

Start conversations with the child and their healthcare providers early—ideally between ages 14 and 16—so the child can be actively involved in the planning process. This is a crucial time for fostering independence.

Review and Update Medical Records:

Ensure that the child's medical records are up-to-date and comprehensive. This includes a detailed medical history, current medications, allergies, treatment plans, and any special instructions for medical procedures or care needs.

Identify Adult Providers:

Research adult care providers who specialize in the child's condition or are comfortable managing complex medical needs. Transitioning to an adult specialist who understands the unique needs of individuals with tracheostomies, feeding tubes, or other chronic conditions is essential.

3. Establishing a Plan for Continued Care

A well-organized care plan is essential to ensure that the child's healthcare needs continue to be met as they transition to adult services.

Create a Comprehensive Care Plan:

Identify Long-Term Healthcare Needs:

Consider all aspects of the child's care, including ongoing treatments, medications, monitoring needs, and follow-up appointments. For children with tracheostomies and feeding tubes, this may include ventilation management, respiratory therapy, and feeding tube monitoring.

Set Goals for the Transition:

The goals of the transition should focus on the child's ability to manage their own care, gradually increasing responsibility over time. This may involve learning to manage their feeding tube, understanding their medications, and becoming involved in decision-making regarding their healthcare.

Build a Support Team:

As the child grows older, they will need a team of healthcare providers who are knowledgeable in adult care as well as the child's specific needs. This may include a primary care physician, specialists (e.g., pulmonologists, gastroenterologists), and a nurse coordinator.

Legal and Financial Considerations:

Depending on the child's condition, they may qualify for specific programs, such as Medicaid or other insurance coverage. Transitioning to adult insurance plans may involve changes in coverage, so it's important to prepare in advance.

Discuss legal issues related to guardianship and consent, especially if the child may not be able to fully manage their healthcare independently. Work with a lawyer if necessary to establish power of attorney or other legal arrangements.

4. Preparing the Child for Increased Independence

The transition to adult care involves not only medical aspects but also the child's increasing independence. It's essential to support the child's emotional and psychological development during this period, helping them gain the skills they need to manage their care more autonomously.

Encourage Self-Care and Autonomy:

Gradually Involve the Child in Their Care:

Start teaching the child how to manage their trach care, G-tube feeding, and other aspects of their medical regimen. Allow them to take on more responsibility over time, with supervision as necessary.

Develop Coping Skills:

Adolescence and young adulthood are critical times for developing coping strategies for managing medical challenges. Encourage the child to participate in social activities, hobbies, and school, and work with a counselor if needed to address any emotional or psychological barriers to independence.

Foster Problem-Solving Skills:

Teach the child how to recognize symptoms of illness or complications, how to troubleshoot issues with their medical devices (e.g., tracheostomy tube or feeding tube), and when to seek help.

5. Addressing Family Dynamics During the Transition

The transition process can be difficult not only for the child but also for the family. It's important to support the family as they navigate the changes and help them adjust to the new reality of adult care.

Communication is Key:

Discuss the Transition Together:

Involve the entire family in discussions about the transition. This may include siblings, parents, and extended family members. Address concerns and expectations as a family unit to ensure everyone is prepared for the changes ahead.

Provide Emotional Support:

The transition can be emotionally challenging for parents, as they may need to let go of some aspects of caregiving. Counseling or support groups for families of children with chronic medical conditions can provide a space for emotional expression and support.

Set Realistic Expectations:

Understand that the transition may not be smooth, and it may take time for both the child and the family to adjust. Being patient and flexible with the process is key to managing this period of change.

6. Resources for Families During the Transition

Numerous resources are available to help families navigate the transition to adult care. These resources can provide guidance, financial assistance, and emotional support.

Types of Resources:

Transition Programs:

Many hospitals and healthcare systems offer transition programs that help guide patients and families through the process of moving from pediatric to adult care. These programs may offer support groups, educational resources, and access to specialized transition coordinators.

Advocacy Groups:

National and local organizations that advocate for individuals with specific medical conditions often have resources for transitioning to adult care. These organizations may provide information on insurance, employment, independent living, and other important topics.

Financial Assistance:

Some families may qualify for government programs, grants, or financial assistance to help cover healthcare costs during the transition. It's important to research options available through local and national resources.

7. Continuing Education and Support

As children with chronic medical conditions transition to adult care, ongoing education is essential. Both the child and their caregivers must remain informed about medical advances, treatment options, and self-care strategies.

Ongoing Learning and Support:

Patient Education:

Ensure that the child continues to receive education about their condition, medications, and any changes in their healthcare needs. The more they understand their condition, the better equipped they will be to manage it.

Support Groups:

Join support groups where individuals with similar conditions can share their experiences and advice. These groups can be invaluable in providing emotional support and practical tips for managing adult care.

Regular Check-Ins with Healthcare Providers:

Continue regular follow-up appointments with healthcare providers to ensure that the transition process is on track and that the child's needs are being met.

8. Conclusion

Transitioning to adult care is a significant step in the life of any child with complex medical needs. With careful planning, ongoing communication, and the right support systems in place, the process can be a smooth and empowering experience. By helping the child gain the skills they need for self-care, addressing family concerns, and ensuring continuity of medical care, families can set the stage for a successful transition to adulthood.

CHAPTER 12

Conclusion and Resources for Ongoing Care

Ensuring Long-Term Success and Support in Pediatric Home Nursing

As you near the end of this guide, it is important to recognize that the journey of pediatric home nursing care for children with complex medical needs, such as tracheostomies and G-tubes, is ongoing. The knowledge, skills, and strategies you've learned in this guide are the foundation for delivering high-quality, compassionate care. However, the road ahead will require continuous learning, adaptation, and support from both the healthcare team and the family. This final chapter focuses on maintaining long-term success in pediatric homecare, as well as offering resources for continued education and assistance.

1. The Ongoing Nature of Pediatric Home Nursing Care

Caring for a child with a tracheostomy or G-tube is a long-term commitment that requires flexibility and perseverance. The medical, emotional, and logistical needs of these children evolve over time, requiring caregivers to adjust their approaches and interventions as the child grows. Pediatric home nursing care is about more than just managing procedures—it's about nurturing the child's development, maintaining family dynamics, and ensuring the child's quality of life.

Key Points to Remember:

- ***Consistency and Stability:*** Maintaining a consistent, stable environment for the child is essential. Routine care, adherence to treatment plans, and a solid relationship with the healthcare team ensure that the child's needs are consistently met.
- ***Continual Assessment:*** The child's health and care needs should be regularly assessed. New challenges will arise as the child grows, and caregivers must stay vigilant and ready to adapt care plans accordingly.

- ***Family Support:*** Pediatric homecare is a team effort that includes not only the healthcare professionals but also the family. The family must be supported emotionally, physically, and psychologically to ensure the child's well-being and to prevent caregiver burnout.

2. Caregiver Self-Care and Support

Caring for a child with complex medical needs can be demanding, both physically and emotionally. It's essential that caregivers take care of themselves in order to provide the best possible care to the child. Support from healthcare professionals, respite care, and regular check-ins with the family can make a significant difference in preventing caregiver burnout.

Strategies for Caregiver Self-Care:

Respite Care:

Arrange for respite care regularly to ensure that caregivers can take breaks and recharge. This may include hiring additional home health aides or asking family members to take over for a few hours.

Build a Support Network:

Connect with other caregivers who have similar experiences. Online support groups, local organizations, and community networks can provide a valuable source of encouragement and advice.

Prioritize Mental Health:

Caregivers should seek professional counseling or therapy if they feel overwhelmed. It is also important to take time for personal activities, such as exercise or hobbies, to maintain emotional well-being.

3. Resources for Ongoing Education and Support

The pediatric homecare landscape is constantly evolving, with new technologies, treatment options, and support strategies emerging regularly. Access to ongoing education and up-to-date resources is vital for both caregivers and healthcare professionals.

Educational Resources for Caregivers:

Home Health Agencies and Providers:

Many agencies provide ongoing training and resources for homecare providers. These may include updated information on tracheostomy care, G-tube management, and emergency protocols.

Online Learning Platforms:

Websites such as Medscape, Nursing Times, and various pediatric homecare provider websites offer free courses and webinars on pediatric care, including specialized care for conditions like tracheostomies and feeding tubes.

Medical Journals and Articles:

Stay informed about the latest medical research and developments related to pediatric homecare by reading journals like Pediatric Nursing and Journal of Pediatric Nursing. These publications often feature evidence-based practices and new care techniques.

Local Hospitals and Medical Centers:

Many hospitals offer continuing education programs for home health nurses and caregivers. These programs may include workshops on advanced nursing skills, pediatric conditions, and family support.

4. Resources for Emotional and Psychological Support

In addition to medical care, emotional and psychological support is crucial for both the child and the family. It's important to have access to mental health resources that can address the stress, anxiety, and other emotional challenges that may arise during long-term care.

Mental Health and Support Resources:

Counseling and Therapy:

Individual or family therapy can provide valuable emotional support. A licensed therapist experienced in working with families of children with special needs can guide families through difficult emotions and communication challenges.

Support Groups:

Connecting with other parents and caregivers through local or online support groups provides a sense of community and shared understanding. Organizations like The National Family Caregivers Association or Family Voices offer connections to local support groups for families dealing with chronic pediatric conditions.

Peer Mentorship Programs:

Some organizations offer peer mentorship programs, where experienced caregivers or parents of children with similar medical needs can offer guidance, practical advice, and emotional support to those just starting the journey of pediatric homecare.

5. Long-Term Care Planning and Transition to Adulthood

As previously discussed, transitioning from pediatric to adult care is an important aspect of long-term planning. The resources and strategies in this chapter can help ensure that children continue to receive the care they need as they grow older.

Planning for Future Medical Needs:

Advanced Directives and Power of Attorney:

As children approach adulthood, it's important to establish advance directives and power of attorney, especially if the child will not be able to make medical decisions independently. This ensures that caregivers and family members have the legal right to make medical decisions on the child's behalf.

Long-Term Care Insurance:

Some families may consider exploring long-term care insurance options to help cover future medical and caregiving needs. Planning ahead for these costs can help alleviate financial stress later on.

6. Conclusion: A Lifelong Commitment to Care

Pediatric home nursing for children with complex medical needs such as tracheostomies and G-tubes is both a deeply rewarding and challenging journey. By maintaining a strong focus on the child's well-being, supporting the family, and continually educating yourself as a caregiver, you help ensure that the child receives the best possible care throughout their life.

Care is not just about procedures—it's about fostering growth, supporting independence, and creating a nurturing environment for the child. Whether you're in the early stages of care or preparing for long-term planning, the goal remains the same: providing a safe, supportive, and loving environment for the child to thrive.

This guide has aimed to provide the tools, resources, and knowledge needed for successful pediatric homecare. But remember, each child's journey is unique, and you'll need to continually adapt and grow with them as their needs evolve.

Thank you for your dedication to providing exceptional care to children with special medical needs. The role you play in their lives is invaluable, and your work makes a significant impact on their health, development, and future.

CHAPTER 13
Ventilator Machines, G-Tube Types, Emergency Management, and Time Management for Homecare Nurses

Providing Specialized Care in the Home Environment: Equipment, Emergencies, and Nurse Self-Care

As a pediatric homecare nurse, your role is multifaceted, requiring you to manage complex medical equipment, respond to emergencies, and balance patient care with your own well-being. This chapter discusses the types of ventilator machines and G-tubes that nurses often work with in the home setting, how to manage during power outages, and strategies for time management, including managing breaks and following agency policies.

1. Types of Ventilator Machines Used in Pediatric Homecare

Ventilators are essential for children with respiratory issues, particularly those with tracheostomies. There are several types of ventilators commonly used in pediatric homecare, each designed for specific respiratory needs. Understanding these devices and how to operate them safely is critical for homecare nurses.

Types of Ventilators:

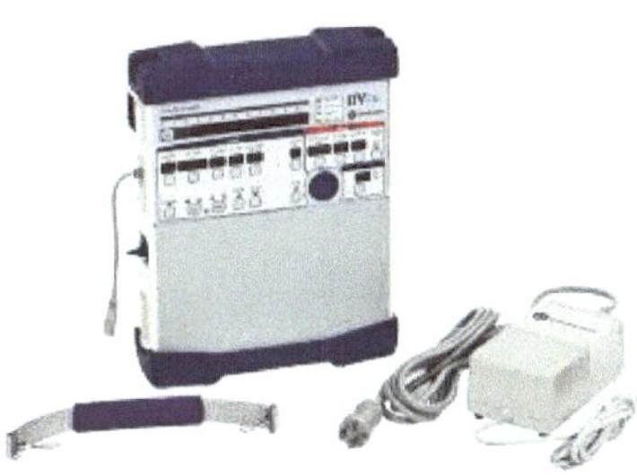

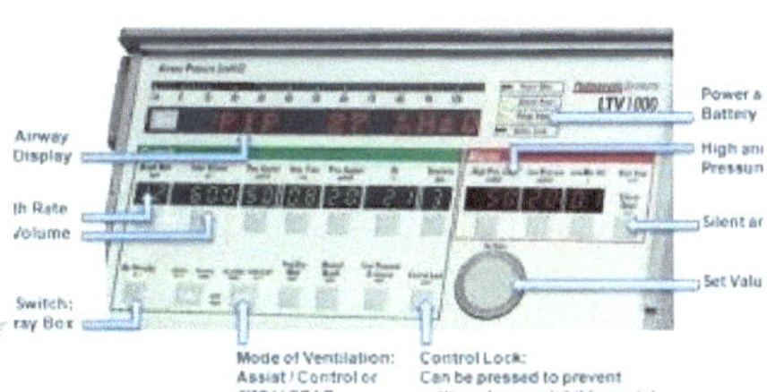

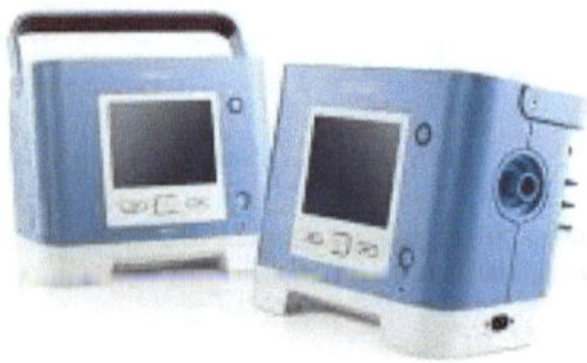

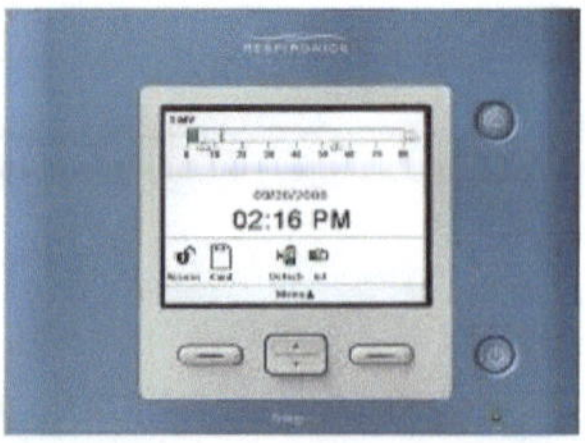

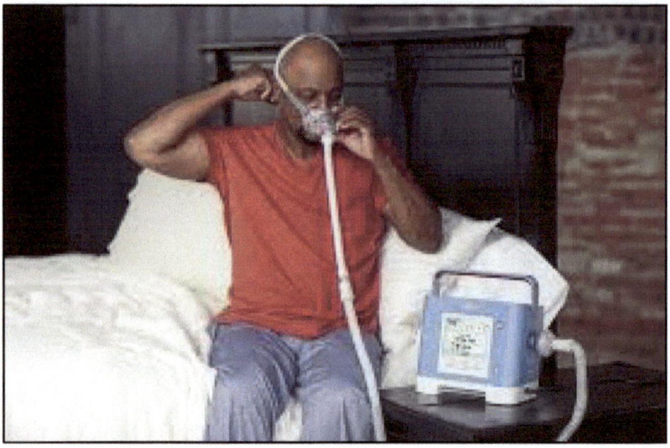

Positive Pressure Ventilators (PPV):

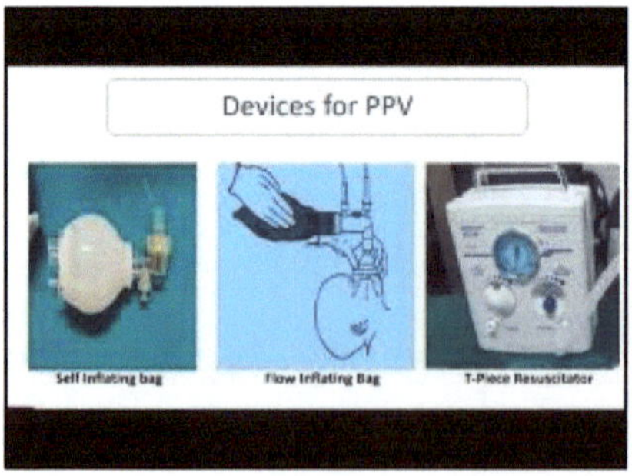

Description: Positive pressure ventilators deliver air into the lungs by increasing the pressure in the airway. These are typically used for patients with conditions such as sleep apnea or chronic respiratory failure.

Examples:

- ***Bilevel Positive Airway Pressure (BiPAP):*** Delivers two levels of pressure (inhalation and exhalation) to help the child breathe more easily.
- ***Continuous Positive Airway Pressure (CPAP):*** Provides a constant flow of air to keep the airways open, commonly used for children with sleep apnea.

Negative Pressure Ventilators:

Description: These devices create negative pressure around the chest wall, aiding in lung expansion. They are less common but may be used for specific conditions.

Example:

The Iron Lung: Though not commonly used today, this device is sometimes found in historical cases where patients require full-body negative pressure support.

Volume-Controlled Ventilators:

Description: These ventilators deliver a set volume of air with each breath, helping to ensure that the child's lungs receive a consistent amount of ventilation.

Example:

Mechanical Ventilators (e.g., LTV series): Used in more critical care situations where precise control over ventilation is needed.

Pressure-Controlled Ventilators:

Description: These ventilators deliver air at a set pressure, which is often used when managing children with conditions that result in compromised lung compliance or resistance.

Ventilator Settings and Monitoring:

Nurses must be proficient in adjusting settings, monitoring alarms, and troubleshooting any issues with the ventilator. This includes checking the tidal volume, respiratory rate, oxygen levels, and ensuring that the airway is clear and the child's comfort is maintained.

2. Types of G-Tubes Used in Pediatric Homecare

A feeding tube, or G-tube, is often required for children who cannot consume food orally. These devices come in different types, each serving specific needs. A homecare nurse must be skilled in managing G-tubes to ensure that feeding and hydration are properly maintained.

Types of G-Tubes:

Standard G-Tube:

Description: A permanent feeding tube is inserted directly into the stomach. It's usually a long-term solution for children who need ongoing nutritional support.

Care: Nurses need to monitor the insertion site for infection, keep the tube clean, and administer feeding as prescribed.

Mic-Key Button:

Description: A low-profile, balloon-retained feeding tube that is less noticeable and is often preferred for children who may need to be more active or mobile.

Care: Mic-Key buttons require careful maintenance to prevent clogging and infection.

PEG Tube (Percutaneous Endoscopic Gastrostomy):

Description: A tube is inserted through the skin into the stomach using an endoscopic procedure. It's commonly used for children with long-term feeding needs.

Care: Nurses monitor for leaks, irritation, and ensure that feeding is done according to prescribed schedules.

Jejunostomy Tube (J-Tube):

Description: A feeding tube that is placed directly into the small intestine (jejunum) rather than the stomach. It's used for children who cannot tolerate stomach feeds due to reflux or delayed gastric emptying.

Care: Requires specialized care to prevent infection and to ensure proper feeding.

Nursing Responsibilities for G-Tube Care:

Nurses must be able to perform daily site care, monitor for infection, handle feeding schedules, and ensure the tube is properly placed. Knowledge of tube replacement protocols and troubleshooting issues like clogged tubes is also essential.

3. Managing Power Outages: Oxygen and Ventilator Care

A sudden power outage in a homecare setting can be a serious concern, particularly for children who rely on ventilators or oxygen machines for their respiratory needs. Nurses must have protocols in place to ensure the child's safety during such events.

Ventilator and Oxygen Management During Power Outages:

Backup Power Source:

Every homecare environment should have an emergency backup power system, such as a battery-powered backup generator or a UPS (Uninterruptible Power Supply) system, that can support ventilators and oxygen concentrators for several hours. Ensure that batteries are regularly charged and in good condition.

Portable Ventilators:

Many modern ventilators come with portable battery packs that can be used during power failures. Nurses must familiarize themselves with these systems and ensure that they are always ready for use in an emergency.

Oxygen Cylinder:

Oxygen tanks are another backup system that can be used if a power failure disrupts an oxygen concentrator. Nurses should have portable oxygen cylinders available, and the family should be trained on how to switch from the concentrator to the cylinder if necessary.

Emergency Preparedness Plan:

Develop and regularly review an emergency preparedness plan with the family, including what to do during a power failure. This should include instructions on using backup power or switching to manual ventilation if necessary, as well as knowing how to call emergency medical services if needed.

4. Managing Lunch Breaks and Nurse Self-Care in Homecare

As a homecare nurse, it can be difficult to balance patient care with the need to take breaks. However, taking a lunch break is essential for maintaining the nurse's health, focus, and ability to provide optimal care. Homecare nurses must also adhere to agency policies when it comes to breaks and self-care.

Lunch Break Strategies for Homecare Nurses:

Follow Agency Policies:

Homecare agencies have specific policies regarding breaks and shift management. Nurses must adhere to these policies to ensure compliance and to provide consistent, high-quality care. This may include guidelines on how to document breaks or ensure that coverage is provided during meal times.

Communicate with the Family:

Communication is essential to ensure that the family understands the nurse's need for a break. The family should be informed in advance about when the nurse will take a break and how the child's care will be managed during that time.

Set Up a Structured Plan:

Nurses should set a clear plan for when and how breaks will occur, and communicate this with the family. This could involve timing the break during a child's nap or quiet time, if possible.

Take Care of Yourself:

Nurses should remember that taking a break not only allows for physical rest but also provides mental clarity to give better care. Having a designated space for breaks and using it effectively is key to reducing burnout and maintaining energy throughout the shift.

5. Time Management During Homecare Shifts

Effective time management is a critical skill for any homecare nurse. With a range of tasks, from performing medical procedures to documenting care, time management helps nurses provide efficient, thorough care.

Time Management Tips:

Prioritize Care Tasks:

Develop a list of tasks and prioritize them based on urgency and importance. This ensures that critical tasks, such as medication administration, G-tube feedings, or ventilator checks, are completed on time.

Plan for Emergencies:

While managing a child with complex medical needs, emergencies may arise. Build extra time into your schedule to handle unforeseen events, whether it's troubleshooting equipment or dealing with a sudden change in the child's condition.

Use Technology for Documentation:

Using digital tools or mobile apps for patient documentation can save time and help keep everything organized. Many homecare agencies offer digital solutions for logging vital signs, medications, and procedures.

Work with the Family:

If appropriate, delegate non-medical tasks to the family members (such as assisting with feeding or preparing meals). This allows you to focus on medical care, while also encouraging family involvement in the care process.

Set Boundaries:

Managing time effectively also means setting boundaries. Clearly define your work hours and break times with the family to avoid interruptions during your scheduled breaks.

6. Conclusion: Effective Homecare Nursing and Self-Care

Managing complex pediatric homecare requires a delicate balance of technical skills, compassion, and time management. As a nurse, you are not only responsible for ensuring the child's medical needs are met but also for taking care of yourself and adhering to agency policies. With the right preparation, clear communication, and effective time management, you can provide exceptional care while maintaining your own well-being.

Remember, you are a vital part of the healthcare team, and your role in supporting the child's health and the family's peace of mind is invaluable.

Here is a template for effective documentation that homecare nurses can use when working with ventilator patients and G-tube care patients. This document ensures comprehensive record-keeping that is both accurate and in line with best practices. It can be used for skilled nursing notes, progress notes, and other required documentation.

Homecare Nurse Skilled Notes for Ventilator and G-Tube Care Patients

Patient Information:

Patient Name: ________________

Date of Birth: ________________

Diagnosis: ________________

Allergies: ________________

Primary Care Physician: ________________

Homecare Agency: ________________

Date of Visit: ________________

Shift: (Morning, Evening, Night) ________________

Nurse Name: ________________

Time In: ________________

Time Out: ________________

1. Ventilator Care

Ventilator Type: ________________

(Example: LTV Series, BiPAP, CPAP, Volume-controlled, Pressure-controlled, etc.)

Ventilator Settings:

Tidal Volume (VT): ________________

Respiratory Rate (RR): ________________

Inspiratory Time (Ti): ________________

Oxygen Concentration (FiO2): ________________

Peak Inspiratory Pressure (PIP): ________________

Positive End-Expiratory Pressure (PEEP): ________________

Other Settings/Adjustments: ________________

Ventilator Functionality:

- **Alarm Settings/Functionality:** (Any alarms noted during the shift – e.g., high pressure, low pressure, apnea, disconnection, etc.)
- **Ventilator Check:** (Check all ventilator components for proper function, including tubing, filters, and humidifier.)
- **Airway management:** (Suctions performed, airway patency checked, secretions documented.)

Patient's Respiratory Status:

Respiratory Rate (RR): ________________

Oxygen Saturation (SpO2): ________________

- **Ventilator Toleration:** (Document any discomfort, distress, or breathing effort observed.)
- **Cough/Secretions:** (Color, consistency, amount of secretions – suction performed as needed.)
- **Signs of Respiratory Distress:** (Labored breathing, tachypnea, use of accessory muscles, cyanosis, etc.)
- **Interventions:** (Include any changes to ventilator settings, suctioning performed, patient repositioning, etc.)

Ventilator Troubleshooting:

(Detail any issues that arose with the ventilator and actions taken to resolve them, including any emergency protocols followed.)

2. G-Tube Care

Type of G-Tube: ________________

(Example: Standard G-tube, Mic-Key Button, PEG tube, J-tube, etc.)

G-Tube Insertion Site:

- **Inspection:** (Describe the appearance of the site: redness, irritation, discharge, swelling, or signs of infection.)
- **Tubing Position:** (Check that the tube is securely in place and not dislodged.)

- **G-Tube Maintenance:** (Cleaning method used, any necessary replacements, or adjustments made.)
- **Other Observations:** (Any additional observations such as leakage, difficulty with feeding, or changes in the site.)

Feeding Plan:

- **Feeding Schedule:** (Document the time and amount of feedings provided, including method: continuous or bolus feeds.)
- **Feeding Solution:** (Type of formula or prescribed nutritional solution, volume administered.)
- **Patient Tolerance:** (Any signs of intolerance such as nausea, vomiting, or discomfort. Document any adverse reactions or complications.)
- **Bowel Movements/Elimination:** (Document frequency, consistency, and any changes in bowel patterns, as well as any concerns.)

Interventions:

- **Tube Flushing:** (Flushing schedule for maintaining patency. Include the amount and type of flush solution used.)
- **G-Tube Replacement:** (If applicable, document any tube replacements, including reason for replacement and patient tolerance.)
- **Complications or Issues Noted:** (Include problems such as tube dislodgement, clogging, leaking, infection, or other concerns.)

3. General Care and Monitoring

Vital Signs: ________________

Heart Rate (HR): ________________

Blood Pressure (BP): ________________

Temperature: ________________

Respiratory Rate (RR): ________________

Oxygen Saturation (SpO2): ________________

Weight (if applicable): (Especially for G-tube patients.) ________________

Skin Integrity:

- **Inspection of Skin:** (Check for signs of pressure ulcers, irritations, or breakdowns around the trach and G-tube sites, including the rest of the body.)
- **Wound Care:** (If applicable, document any dressing changes or treatments for wounds.)

Pain Management:

Pain Assessment: (Any complaints of pain or discomfort noted. Use pain scale if appropriate, and document any pain interventions provided.)

Patient Activity:

- **Positioning/Movement:** (Include any repositioning done during the shift. Document patient activity tolerance and mobility.)
- **Physical Therapy or Rehabilitative Activities:** (If applicable, any activities or movements encouraged or performed to improve health or prevent complications.)

4. Nurse's Observations and Plan of Care:

Patient's Condition/Progress:

(Describe any significant changes, improvements, or declines in the patient's condition, particularly in respiratory function, nutrition, or overall well-being.)

Plan of Care for Next Shift:

- **Interventions Needed:** (Specific care or medical interventions required for the next shift.)
- **Follow-up:** (Any follow-up actions needed, such as physician contact, adjustments to ventilator settings, or further assessments of the G-tube site.)

Family or Caregiver Instructions:

(If applicable, document any instructions provided to family members or caregivers regarding patient care, ventilator management, or G-tube maintenance.)

Nurse's Signature: ________________

Date and Time: ________________

5. Emergency Protocols (if applicable):

Ventilator or G-Tube Emergency:

- **Actions Taken in Emergency:** (Detail any emergency protocols followed, including equipment troubleshooting, patient stabilization, and emergency contacts made.)
- **Outcome:** (Patient's response to interventions during the emergency.)

6. Nurse's Breaks:

(Ensure this section is filled in accordance with the homecare agency's break policy.)

Break Taken: (Document if and when a break was taken during the shift. Breaks must be scheduled according to agency policy, and patient care should remain uninterrupted.)

7. Sign-Off by Supervisor/Agency (if applicable):

Supervisor's Name: ________________

Comments: ________________

Signature/Date: ________________

This documentation ensures that all aspects of care are covered comprehensively, including both routine tasks and emergency protocols, while helping homecare nurses stay compliant with agency policies.

After receiving training in tracheostomy and G-tube care, a novice nurse can effectively market herself in job applications and resumes by focusing on relevant skills, certifications, and practical knowledge gained during training. Below are strategies for presenting oneself as a qualified candidate:

1. Craft a Strong Summary or Objective Statement

The objective or professional summary at the top of the resume should highlight key skills, certifications, and a passion for pediatric homecare nursing. This is where the nurse can emphasize her newly acquired expertise in tracheostomy and G-tube care.

Example Summary: "Compassionate and detail-oriented Registered Nurse (RN) with recent specialized training in pediatric tracheostomy and G-tube care. Committed to providing high-quality, patient-centered care in the home environment, focusing on respiratory management, feeding tube support, and overall patient comfort. Eager to bring clinical expertise and a dedication to improving patient outcomes to a homecare nursing role."

2. Highlight Relevant Skills and Certifications

List all technical skills and certifications acquired during training, making them easily identifiable to hiring managers. Include both hard and soft skills that demonstrate competence in pediatric care.

Example Skills Section:

Tracheostomy Care:

- Suctioning, cleaning, and changing tracheostomy tubes
- Managing respiratory distress and ensuring airway patency
- Monitoring ventilator settings and alarms

G-Tube Care:

- Insertion site inspection, cleaning, and maintenance
- Administering feedings via G-tube (bolus and continuous)
- Flushing tubes and troubleshooting common G-tube issues
- Pediatric CPR and Basic Life Support (BLS) Certified

Patient Education: Empowering families to care for their loved ones with tracheostomies and G-tubes

Compassionate Communication: Building trust with families and patients to ensure comfort and safety

3. Focus on Practical Experience and Clinical Training

Even as a novice nurse, if training was hands-on, include those details to demonstrate practical experience. If there was any direct care, shadowing, or internships with pediatric tracheostomy and G-tube patients, be sure to mention it.

Example Experience Section:

Pediatric Homecare Nursing Intern

ABC Homecare Agency | City, State

Month Year – Month Year

- Assisted in the care of pediatric patients with tracheostomies, including daily suctioning, airway maintenance, and monitoring ventilator settings.
- Provided G-tube care, including administration of feedings, tube flushing, and inspection for infection.
- Collaborated with a team of healthcare providers to monitor patients' progress and adjust care plans as needed.
- Trained family members on tracheostomy and G-tube care, ensuring they understood safety protocols and emergency procedures.

4. Include Any Related Continuing Education or Certification

If the nurse has taken additional courses (e.g., tracheostomy care, pediatric advanced life support, etc.), be sure to list them. This shows a commitment to professional growth and up-to-date skills.

Example Continuing Education:

- **Advanced Pediatric Tracheostomy Care Training**
  Institution Name | Month Year
- **G-Tube Management and Feeding Techniques**
  Institution Name | Month Year

5. Use Keywords and Phrases for Applicant Tracking Systems (ATS)

Many employers use ATS to screen resumes before they are even seen by a recruiter. To pass through these systems, ensure the resume uses relevant keywords. Include terms like:

- Pediatric homecare
- Tracheostomy care
- G-tube management
- Ventilator support

- Patient education
- Feeding tube care

6. Leverage Volunteer or Personal Experience (if applicable)

If the nurse has any volunteer experience or personal caregiving experience related to tracheostomy or G tube care, this can be included as well. While not professional experience, it can still show a deep understanding and hands-on ability.

Example Volunteer Experience:

Volunteer Caregiver for Pediatric Tracheostomy Patient

Private Residence | City, State

Month Year – Present

- Assisted with daily tracheostomy care, including cleaning, suctioning, and monitoring respiratory status.
- Provided G-tube feedings and educated family members on proper G-tube care techniques.

7. Show Enthusiasm and a Willingness to Learn

Novice nurses should emphasize their eagerness to continue learning and growing in the field. Employers value nurses who show initiative, even if they don't have years of experience yet.

Example Cover Letter Excerpt:

"I am excited about the opportunity to apply my recent training in pediatric tracheostomy and G-tube care to contribute to your team. My hands-on experience, combined with my passion for pediatric nursing, drives me to continually improve my skills and make a positive impact in the lives of patients and their families."

8. Provide References or Testimonials

If possible, include references from instructors, clinical preceptors, or family members who can speak to your competence in pediatric care, tracheostomy, and G-tube management. This helps to bolster your credibility as a new nurse entering the field.

Example Resume Format:

Name

Contact Information

Phone | Email | LinkedIn (if applicable)

Objective:

[Include your tailored professional summary or objective]

Education:

Registered Nurse (RN), [School Name, Graduation Date]

Certifications:

- Basic Life Support (BLS)
- Advanced Pediatric Life Support (APLS) (if applicable)
- Advanced Pediatric Tracheostomy Care Training
- G-Tube Management and Feeding Techniques

Skills:

- Tracheostomy and Ventilator Management
- Pediatric Homecare Nursing
- G-Tube Feeding and Maintenance
- Family Education and Support
- Patient Documentation and Care Plans

Experience:

Pediatric Homecare Nursing Intern

[Agency Name, Location]

[Dates]

[List key responsibilities, focusing on tracheostomy and G-tube care]

Volunteer Caregiver for Pediatric Tracheostomy Patient

[Location, Dates]

[List duties related to G-tube and trach care]

References:

Available upon request or [list references here, if applicable].

By strategically showcasing these skills, training, and experiences, the novice nurse can create a resume and application that not only highlights her qualifications but also her passion and readiness to work in pediatric homecare settings.

Skilled Nursing Note – Pediatric Tracheostomy & G-Tube Care Template

Patient Name: ____________________________

DOB: ___________ MRN: ___________

Date: ___________

Shift: [ ] Day (0700–1900) [ ] Night (1900–0700)

Nurse Name/Title: ____________________________

Subjective:

Patient verbal / ☐ Non-verbal

Baseline behavior/interaction: ___________________________________

Parent/caregiver report: ____

Objective:

Airway/Respiratory:

Trach type/size: ___________________

Trach status: ☐ Patent ☐ Obstructed ☐ Dislodged

Site appearance: ☐ Clean/dry ☐ Red ☐ Drainage (describe):________

Suctioning: ☐ Required ☐ Not required - Times: _______

Secretion color/consistency: ____________________

Humidification: ☐ Trach collar ☐ HME ☐ Other: ___________

O2 delivery: ☐ Room air ☐ O2 ______ L/min Sat range: ___%

Respiratory effort: ☐ Normal ☐ Labored ☐ Retractions

☐ Nasal flaring

Gastrointestinal/Nutrition:

G-tube type: _______________

Site status: ☐ Intact ☐ Red ☐ Leaking ☐ Other: ____________

Feeding method: ☐ Bolus ☐ Continuous

Volume: _________ Type: ____________________

Tolerance: ☐ Good ☐ Residuals present ☐ Vomiting ☐ Other: ____

Flushes: ______ mL sterile water ☐ Pre ☐ Post ☐ Both

Meds given via G-tube: ☐ Yes ☐ No List: ______________________

Skin Integrity:

Repositioned q___h

Diaper area: ☐ Clear ☐ Red ☐ Breakdown

Pressure areas: ☐ Intact ☐ At risk ☐ Breakdown (location): _________

Activity/Interaction:

Asleep ☐ Awake ☐ Tolerated handling

Activities completed: ____

Sleep/Comfort (Night Shift):

Restful sleep ☐ Frequent waking ☐ Required intervention (describe): ________

Assessment:

Patient stable ☐ Change in condition (describe): ____________________

Summary of response to care: ______________________________________

Plan:

- Continue trach and G-tube care per protocol
- Monitor respiratory status, site integrity, and feeding tolerance
- Reinforce caregiver education (if applicable)
- Notify MD/NP if changes occur

Signature/Title: ___________________________Date/Time: ____________

Your documentation format will depend on the protocols or regulations of your Homecare agency.

SCENARIO: A Typical 7 AM - 7 PM Homecare Nurse Shift

Patient Profile:

Name: Alex

Age: 3 years old

Diagnosis: Tracheostomy, G-tube, and Complex Respiratory Issues

Ventilator Support: Yes, on bilevel positive airway pressure (BiPAP) at night

Feeding Method: G-tube, formula feeds

Time In: 7:00 AM

Time Out: 7:00 PM

Shift Duration: 12 hours

7:00 AM - Arrival and Handoff

- **Arrive at the Home:** The nurse arrives promptly at 7:00 AM. Before starting care, she reviews Alex's medical records and speaks with the night shift nurse for a detailed handoff. The night nurse mentions that Alex had a stable night, with no major concerns, but reports some mild coughing during the early morning hours.
- **Prepare Equipment:** The nurse checks Alex's equipment to ensure everything is functioning, including the ventilator, oxygen supply, and feeding pump. She verifies that emergency supplies (such as a spare trach tube and suctioning equipment) are readily available.

7:15 AM - Initial Assessment and Vital Signs

- **Patient Check:** The nurse approaches Alex's room quietly to avoid waking him. Alex is sleeping in his crib, and his ventilator is running as prescribed.
- **Vital Signs:**
  - **Heart Rate:** 110 bpm
  - **Respiratory Rate:** 20 breaths per minute
  - **Oxygen Saturation (SpO2):** 94% (on CPAP)
  - **Temperature:** 98.6°F

- Blood Pressure: 85/55 mmHg

- **Tracheostomy Check:** The nurse inspects Alex's tracheostomy site for signs of infection or irritation. There are no abnormalities, and the trach is secure.
- **Ventilator Settings:** She confirms the ventilator settings are appropriate, with bilevel positive airway pressure (BiPAP) for comfort and ventilation support.

7:45 AM - Suctioning and Respiratory Care

- **Suctioning:** The nurse performs gentle suctioning on Alex's trach tube to clear any mucus or secretions. She ensures that the suctioning procedure is sterile to prevent any risk of infection.
- **Secretions:** There is a moderate amount of mucus, which is successfully cleared.
- **Post-Suctioning Check:** After suctioning, the nurse listens to Alex's lungs to assess his respiratory status. No wheezing or signs of distress are noted.

8:00 AM - G-Tube Care and Feeding

- **G-Tube Inspection:** The nurse inspects Alex's G-tube site for any redness, irritation, or leakage. The site looks healthy with no signs of infection.
- **Feeding Preparation:** The nurse prepares Alex's formula according to the prescribed schedule and ensures the feeding tube is patent. She prepares a bolus feeding.
- **G-Tube Feeding:** Alex's feeding is administered via the G-tube, with the nurse monitoring the flow and ensuring no complications during the feeding.
- **Feeding Tolerance:** Alex tolerates the feeding well, and the nurse watches for any signs of nausea, bloating, or discomfort.

9:00 AM - Family Communication and Education

- **Family Interaction:** The nurse takes some time to discuss Alex's care plan with his parents. She explains how to perform daily trach care, proper techniques for G-tube feeding, and how to recognize signs of infection or complications with the trach and G-tube.

- **Emergency Protocols:** The nurse provides a refresher on emergency procedures, such as what to do if the trach becomes dislodged or if there are signs of feeding intolerance.
- **Patient Education:** The nurse walks the parents through the proper way to flush the G-tube after feedings and how to handle the equipment.

<u>10:00 AM</u> - Repositioning and Comfort Measures

- **Repositioning:** To prevent pressure sores and improve comfort, the nurse carefully repositions Alex in bed, checking for signs of discomfort, pressure points, or skin breakdown.
- **Comfort Checks:** Alex appears comfortable, and the nurse ensures he is well-supported with pillows for optimal positioning.
- **Routine Checks:** She checks his vitals again, and everything remains stable. She also adjusts his blankets to ensure he is not too warm or too cold.

<u>10:30 AM</u> - Nurse's Break and Equipment Check

- **Nurse Break:** The nurse takes a 15-minute break, allowing the family to take over basic monitoring of Alex's condition. During this time, the nurse checks the backup equipment to ensure it is working properly (spare trach tubes, suction device, etc.).
- **Equipment Status:** She tests the portable suction unit to ensure it's charged and functioning, in case of an emergency transport situation.

<u>11:00 AM</u> - Second Feeding and Medication Administration

- **G-Tube Feeding:** It's time for Alex's second scheduled feeding. The nurse follows the same procedure as earlier, preparing the formula, administering it via the G-tube, and monitoring for signs of feeding intolerance.
- **Medications:** Alex's prescribed medications for the day are given through the G-tube with a small amount of water to flush the line.
- **Post-Feeding Monitoring:** After the feeding, the nurse ensures that Alex is positioned correctly to allow for digestion and minimize the risk of aspiration.

12:00 PM - Lunch Break and Documentation

- **Lunch Break:** The nurse takes her lunch break, ensuring that Alex's parents are aware of the feeding schedule and emergency procedures during this time.
- **Documentation:** She completes her documentation for the first part of the shift, noting all interventions, including vital signs, suctioning, G-tube feeding, medications administered, and family interactions.

1:00 PM - Afternoon Care and Tracheostomy Care

- **Tracheostomy Care:** The nurse performs a more detailed trach care routine, cleaning the trach tube, changing the inner cannula (if needed), and applying a clean dressing to the site. She ensures that the site is dry and free of any infection.
- **Ventilator Check:** The nurse checks the ventilator settings once more and confirms that everything is functioning properly. She also checks the air humidifier and filters to ensure optimal conditions for breathing.

2:00 PM - Monitoring and Assessment

- **Patient Monitoring:** The nurse continues to monitor Alex's condition closely, ensuring that all vital signs are within normal ranges. She checks his SpO2 levels again (95%) and adjusts his ventilator settings slightly, as per the physician's orders, to ensure optimal breathing.
- **Observations:** Alex is resting comfortably with no signs of distress. His skin remains intact, and there are no signs of discomfort around the G-tube or trach.

3:00 PM - Family Education and Support

- **Family Interaction:** The nurse continues to work closely with Alex's parents, reinforcing training on caring for the trach tube and G-tube, as well as recognizing warning signs of potential complications.
- **Emergency Drills:** The nurse leads a brief emergency drill with the family, explaining how to act if the trach tube becomes dislodged or if Alex shows signs of respiratory distress.

4:30 PM - Repositioning and Comfort Checks

- **Repositioning:** Alex is repositioned again to avoid any pressure on his body and ensure comfort. The nurse checks the alignment of his body and adjusts his pillows for optimal posture.
- **Vital Signs:** A final round of vital checks is conducted. No new concerns are noted, and Alex remains stable.

6:00 PM - Preparation for Handoff

- **Final Assessment:** The nurse reviews the shift's activities, including all care interventions, vitals, and family education. She prepares a detailed report for the evening nurse, outlining the ventilator settings, feeding schedule, and any concerns that may need attention during the night shift.
- **Family Handoff:** The nurse updates the family about Alex's care plan for the next 12 hours and provides any last-minute instructions regarding feeding or emergency procedures.

7:00 PM - End of Shift

Time Out: The nurse formally ends her shift, documenting any final notes and preparing the room for the evening nurse's arrival. She ensures that Alex is in a comfortable position, with his ventilator set properly and all necessary supplies in place.

Key Takeaways:

- **Comprehensive Care:** Throughout the 12-hour shift, the nurse ensures all aspects of Alex's care are addressed, from ventilator checks and suctioning to G-tube feedings and family education.
- **Family Support:** The nurse provides continuous education and emotional support to the family, empowering them to care for Alex confidently.
- **Documentation and Communication:** The nurse maintains accurate and detailed documentation, ensuring continuity of care and clear communication for the next shift.

This scenario demonstrates the nurse's ability to balance complex medical tasks with supportive family education and patient-centered care over a full 12-hour shift.

SCENARIO: A Typical 7 PM - 7 AM Homecare Nurse Night Shift

Patient Profile:

Name: Mia

Age: 2 years old

Diagnosis: Tracheostomy, G-tube, Chronic Respiratory Issues, and Recurrent Aspiration Pneumonia

Ventilator Support: Yes, on BiPAP (Bilevel Positive Airway Pressure) overnight

Feeding Method: G-tube for feeding and hydration

Time In: 7:00 PM

Time Out: 7:00 AM

Shift Duration: 12 hours

7:00 PM - Arrival and Handoff

- **Arrival at the Home:** The nurse arrives at Mia's home and reviews her medical records. Mia's parents provide a thorough handoff, mentioning any concerns from the day shift and informing the nurse about Mia's current condition. Mia had a stable day but was a little fussy after her evening feeding.
- **Equipment Check:** The nurse checks Mia's equipment to ensure everything is functioning, including her BiPAP machine, oxygen support, suction device, G-tube, and ventilator. She verifies that all alarms are set properly on the equipment.

7:15 PM - Initial Assessment and Vital Signs

- **Patient Check:** The nurse approaches Mia's crib quietly as she is resting, with her BiPAP in place. Mia's parents confirm she is asleep, and the nurse proceeds with a quick assessment.
- **Vital Signs:**
  - **Heart Rate:** 108 bpm
  - **Respiratory Rate:** 16 breaths per minute
  - **Oxygen Saturation (SpO2):** 96% (on BiPAP)

    - **Temperature:** 98.2°F
    - **Blood Pressure:** 85/55 mmHg
- **Tracheostomy and BiPAP Check:** The nurse inspects Mia's tracheostomy site for signs of infection and ensures her BiPAP machine is running correctly. The settings are confirmed: Inspiratory Pressure of 12 cmH2O and Expiratory Pressure of 6 cmH2O.

<u>7:45 PM</u> - Suctioning and Respiratory Care

- **Suctioning:** The nurse performs gentle suctioning of Mia's trach to clear any secretions that may have accumulated during the day. Mia's respiratory rate remains stable, and her lungs are clear after suctioning.
- **Secretions:** Minimal secretions are noted, and the suctioning process is completed without complications.
- **Airway Monitoring:** After suctioning, the nurse ensures Mia's trach tube remains secure and that the airway is clear. She checks for any irritation or discomfort around the trach site.

<u>8:00 PM</u> - G-Tube Feeding and Medication

- **G-Tube Care:** The nurse inspects Mia's G-tube insertion site, noting that there is no redness, leakage, or irritation.
- **Prepare Feeding:** Mia's evening formula is prepared according to her prescribed feeding plan, and the nurse sets the G-tube for bolus feeding.
- **Feeding Administration:** The nurse delivers the formula via the G-tube, monitoring Mia's comfort throughout the process.
- **Feeding Tolerance:** Mia tolerates the feeding without issue, and there are no signs of discomfort or vomiting.
- **Medications:** Mia's prescribed medications are administered via the G-tube as per her schedule. The nurse uses a small amount of water to flush the tube after each medication.

<u>8:45 PM</u> - Family Communication and Update

- **Family Check-In:** The nurse updates Mia's parents on her condition. She discusses how the day shift went, addresses any concerns from the family, and answers questions regarding Mia's tracheostomy care, feeding schedule, or equipment usage.

- **Emergency Protocols:** The nurse reviews emergency protocols for trach tube dislodgement or respiratory distress, ensuring the parents are comfortable with the steps to take in case of an emergency.

9:00 PM - Nurse's Break and Equipment Check

- **Break:** The nurse takes a 15 minute break, allowing the family to monitor Mia while she rests. During this time, the nurse checks all backup equipment, ensuring everything is in good working order. She confirms that there is a spare trach tube, suction devices, oxygen tanks, and any necessary supplies readily available.
- **Backup Checks:** The nurse tests the portable suction unit to ensure it's fully charged and functioning in case of an emergency.

9:30 PM - Positioning and Comfort

- **Repositioning:** The nurse gently repositions Mia in her crib to ensure that her body is properly supported and aligned. This helps prevent pressure sores and promotes comfort while she sleeps.
- **Comfort Monitoring:** Mia's body is checked for any signs of discomfort or pressure points. Her blankets are adjusted to ensure she is not too warm or cold.

10:00 PM - Monitoring and Documentation

- **Ongoing Monitoring:** The nurse continues to monitor Mia's BiPAP settings and oxygen saturation levels throughout the night. Mia's vitals remain stable, and she shows no signs of respiratory distress.
- **Documentation:** The nurse documents all care provided, including suctioning, G-tube feeding, medication administration, and patient assessments. She also notes any family education provided during the shift.

12:00 AM - Midnight Checks and Assessment

- **Routine Checks:** The nurse performs a round of vital checks, ensuring that Mia's heart rate, respiratory rate, and oxygen saturation remain within normal limits. No changes are noted, and Mia remains comfortably asleep.

- **Tracheostomy Care:** The nurse performs a more detailed trach care routine, cleaning the inner cannula (if needed), changing the trach dressing, and ensuring the site remains clean and free from infection.

2:00 AM - G-Tube Feeding and Care

- **Second G-Tube Feeding:** It's time for Mia's next scheduled feeding. The nurse prepares the formula and delivers it via the G-tube.
- **Feeding Process:** Mia is positioned slightly upright during the feeding to reduce the risk of aspiration. The nurse monitors her tolerance, ensuring that there are no signs of discomfort.
- **Medication Administration:** After the feeding, the nurse administers any scheduled medications, flushing the G-tube afterward to prevent clogging.

3:00 AM - Family Support and Break

- **Family Support:** The nurse speaks with Mia's parents, providing emotional support and answering any questions they may have. She reaffirms the importance of observing Mia's breathing closely and provides guidance on suctioning or G-tube care if they need to take over during the nurse's break.
- **Break:** The nurse takes another 15-minute break, during which Mia's parents monitor her condition.

4:00 AM - Comfort and Monitoring

- **Positioning:** The nurse checks Mia's comfort again, ensuring that she is positioned well and has no pressure points on her body. Mia's condition remains stable, and she is resting comfortably.
- **Ongoing Monitoring:** The nurse continues to check her vital signs and respiratory status every hour, documenting any changes or concerns in her chart.

6:00 AM - Final Check and Handoff Preparation

- **Morning Assessment:** As the shift comes to a close, the nurse conducts a final assessment of Mia's condition, ensuring that all medical equipment is functioning and that Mia remains stable.
- **Vital Signs:**
  - **Heart Rate:** 110 bpm

- **Respiratory Rate:** 18 breaths per minute
- **SpO2:** 95% (on BiPAP)

- **Prepare for Handoff:** The nurse prepares a comprehensive report for the incoming nurse, detailing Mia's condition, equipment settings, and any concerns or changes in her care throughout the shift. She ensures that all necessary information is provided to ensure continuity of care.

7:00 AM - End of Shift

Time Out: The nurse formally ends her shift, ensuring that Mia is comfortable and all necessary supplies are ready for the next shift. She gives a final update to the family, reassuring them that Mia's condition is stable and providing any instructions for the next nurse.

Key Takeaways:

- **Patient Safety and Monitoring:** Throughout the 12-hour night shift, the nurse provides consistent care, checking Mia's respiratory status, G-tube feedings, and overall comfort.
- **Family Education and Communication:** The nurse communicates regularly with Mia's parents, providing education and emotional support, ensuring they are confident in managing the care during off-hours.
- **Attention to Detail and Documentation:** The nurse meticulously documents all care activities, ensuring that every intervention is recorded and that Mia's condition is accurately monitored.

This scenario illustrates the responsibilities and care processes a homecare nurse would undertake during a night shift with a pediatric patient requiring ventilator and G-tube support.

Here are some organizations in the U.S. that offer training for tracheostomy and ventilator care as well as G-tube care:

1. American Association for Respiratory Care (AARC)

Services: The AARC offers courses, webinars, and certifications related to respiratory care, including ventilator management and tracheostomy care.

Website: www.aarc.org

2. National Association for Homecare & Hospice (NAHC)

Services: NAHC provides training programs and certifications on a variety of home healthcare topics, including tracheostomy care, ventilator management, and G-tube care for pediatric patients.

Website: www.nahc.org

3. Pediatric Home Service

Services: Pediatric Home Service offers specialized training for nurses and caregivers on tracheostomy care, ventilator use, and G-tube management for children with complex needs.

Website: www.pediatrichomeservice.com

4. The National Tracheostomy Safety Project

Services: This organization provides resources and training focused on safe tracheostomy care and the management of pediatric and adult patients with tracheostomies.

Website: www.tracheostomy.com

5. Ventilator-Assisted Children's Home Program (VACH)

Services: VACH offers comprehensive training for healthcare providers on ventilator management and care for children who require respiratory support. It includes tracheostomy care and G-tube feeding education.

Website: www.choc.org

6. Breathe California

Services: Breathe California offers training for caregivers and healthcare professionals, focusing on respiratory issues, tracheostomy care, and G-tube management.

Website: www.breathecalifornia.org

7. Lincare

Services: Lincare provides respiratory care training for healthcare professionals, including tracheostomy and ventilator management. They offer resources for caregivers to learn about G-tube care as well.

Website: www.lincare.com

8. Infusion Nurses Society (INS)

Services: The INS offers training and certifications for nurses in infusion therapy, which includes G-tube management and education on feeding tube care.

Website: www.ins1.org

9. The American Lung Association

Services: The American Lung Association provides educational materials and training on various respiratory care topics, including tracheostomy care and ventilator management.

Website: www.lung.org

10. Homecare University (by BAYADA Home Health Care)

Services: BAYADA's Homecare University offers training on pediatric homecare, including tracheostomy and ventilator management, and G-tube care, with online courses and resources for caregivers.

Website: www.bayada.com

These organizations provide valuable resources, online courses, and certifications to help healthcare professionals and caregivers gain the necessary skills for managing pediatric patients with tracheostomies, ventilators, and G-tubes.

Here's a sample reference page for your book based on the chapters you've worked on so far, including the organizations mentioned for training in tracheostomy, ventilator, and G-tube care:

Pediatric Homecare Nurse Guide to Annual Skills Reviews

Annual skills reviews are essential for maintaining clinical excellence and ensuring that pediatric homecare nurses remain proficient in the specialized care they provide. These reviews also align with regulatory and agency standards for competency, safety, and quality care.

Purpose of Annual Skills Review

- Verify continued competence in critical nursing procedures.
- Update skills based on new equipment, procedures, or best practices.
- Reinforce knowledge of agency protocols and care standards.
- Meet compliance with state, federal, and accreditation requirements.

Core Competencies Typically Reviewed

Airway Management & Tracheostomy Care

- Suctioning technique (sterile vs. clean)
- Tracheostomy tube change (emergency and routine)
- Stoma site care and infection control
- Emergency response to decannulation

Gastrostomy (G-Tube) Care

- Tube site cleaning and maintenance
- Feeding procedures (bolus and continuous)
- Troubleshooting common issues (e.g., clogs, leakage)
- G-tube replacement protocols (per facility policy)

Ventilator & Oxygen Use

- Ventilator settings understanding and documentation
- Circuit and humidification care
- Emergency bagging and equipment failure protocols
- Oxygen cylinder safety and backup systems

Medication Administration

- Safe medication prep and delivery via the enteral route

- Understanding compatibility with feeding formulas
- Time-sensitive medication reminders and documentation

Infection Control & Universal Precautions

- Hand hygiene, PPE, and safe disposal
- Preventing hospital-acquired infections at home
- Isolation procedures when necessary

Documentation and Reporting

- Accurate, skilled nursing notes
- Incident reporting
- Communication with physicians and interdisciplinary team

Patient & Family Education

- Teaching family members to participate in care
- Demonstrating emergency response techniques
- Promoting developmental and emotional support

Time Management and Shift Organization

- Prioritizing care
- Managing feeding, med schedules, and therapies
- Break coverage planning

How to Prepare for Your Annual Review

- Review your agency's skill checklist ahead of time.
- Request refreshers or simulations on skills you feel less confident in.
- Bring questions or cases you encountered for discussion.
- Update any certifications required (BLS, PALS, etc.).

Documentation

Nurses must sign off on each skill competency under observation by a clinical supervisor or educator. These are typically kept in the nurse's personnel file for audit and quality review.

Here's a printable one-page checklist version of the Pediatric Homecare Nurse Guide to Annual Skills Reviews. You can copy this into a document or print as is:

Annual Skills Review Checklist for Pediatric Homecare Nurses

Nurse Name: ______________________ Date: ______________

Supervisor/Evaluator: ______________________

Agency: ______________________

1. Airway Management & Tracheostomy Care

- Suctioning (Sterile/Clean technique)
- Routine tracheostomy tube change
- Emergency trach change procedure
- Stoma site care
- Response to accidental decannulation
- Trach tie changes and safety check

2. Gastrostomy (G-Tube) Care

- Site assessment and cleaning
- Bolus feeding procedure
- Continuous feeding pump setup
- G-tube troubleshooting (leaks, clogs)
- Emergency tube dislodgement protocol
- G-tube change procedure (if permitted by policy)

3. Ventilator & Oxygen Use

- Ventilator function review
- Circuit setup and humidifier maintenance
- Oxygen tank usage and safety
- Manual resuscitation (bagging)
- Backup equipment procedures
- Power outage protocol

4. Medication Administration

- Med prep and administration via G-tube

- Medication/fluid compatibility checks
- Accurate timing and dose verification
- Documentation of med administration

5. Infection Control & Universal Precautions

- Proper hand hygiene
- Use of gloves, masks, gowns
- Equipment and supply sanitation
- Disposal of biohazard waste
- Isolation protocol (when applicable)

6. Documentation and Reporting

- Completion of shift notes
- Incident reporting (falls, trach events)
- Communication with care team
- Documentation of parent teaching

7. Patient & Family Education

- Teaching care routines to family
- Demonstrating suctioning/trach care
- Emergency response training
- Reinforcing safe handling and positioning

8. Time Management

- Shift organization and planning
- Feeding/medication schedule tracking
- Prioritizing skilled nursing tasks
- Taking appropriate breaks per policy

Evaluator Comments:

Nurse Signature: ________________Evaluator Signature:_________________

Here's a practical list of personal and professional items that day shift and night shift pediatric homecare nurses should bring on the job. These ensure comfort, preparedness, and compliance with both clinical and agency standards.

Professional Items (Essential for Both Shifts)

Nursing Bag or Backpack with:

- Stethoscope (pediatric-size preferred)
- Pulse oximeter (if not provided at home)
- Blood pressure cuff (manual and/or digital, pediatric size)
- Thermometer
- Medical scissors and tape
- Penlight
- Hand sanitizer and gloves (if agency doesn't supply)
- Spare PPE (mask, gown, eye shield)
- Alcohol wipes and saline flushes
- Documentation tools (clipboard, notebook, care log sheets)

Paperwork & Reference Materials

- Patient care plan
- Agency protocol binder or quick guide
- Medication list (if permitted to bring)
- Emergency contact list

Badge and Licensure

- Photo ID badge
- RN/LPN license copy (some agencies require)
- CPR/PALS certification card

Technology

- Charged cell phone (for emergencies and documentation apps)
- Agency-issued tablet or laptop (if applicable)
- Backup charging cable/power bank

Personal Items – Day Shift

- Light jacket or sweater (home temps vary)
- Water bottle (hydration is key!)
- Healthy snacks or lunch (easy-to-eat options, especially if the child needs constant observation)

- Coffee/tea travel mug
- Breath mints or gum
- Extra scrubs or undershirt (in case of soiling)
- Small notebook/journal for notes or time tracking

Personal Items – Night Shift

- Quiet snacks (protein bars, fruit, etc.)
- Blanket or light throw (if permitted to rest during stable hours)
- Eye drops or lip balm (for dry home environments)
- A Thermos with a warm drink
- Book or light reading (if appropriate during downtime)
- Comfort items (neck pillow, compression socks)
- Extra batteries or flashlight (for low-light monitoring)

Optional but Helpful for Both Shifts

- Mini whiteboard (for quick reminders or med times)
- Watch with a second hand (for accurate assessments)
- Small calendar or planner
- Agency policy manual or cheat sheet
- Personal hygiene kit (toothbrush, deodorant, hand lotion)

Several homecare agencies and training providers in the U.S. offer tracheostomy care courses for nurses. These programs are designed to enhance the skills of homecare nurses in managing tracheostomy and ventilator-dependent patients. Here are some notable options:

1. Journey University – Comprehensive Training for Homecare Nurses

- **Format:** Online course
- **Overview:** Provides foundational knowledge in tracheostomy and ventilator care, including ventilator settings, suctioning techniques, and emergency management.
- **Ideal for:** Homecare nurses seeking to build or refresh their skills in tracheostomy and ventilator management.
- **More information:** journeyuniversity.tovuti.io

2. MedBridge – Tracheostomy Care Course

- **Format:** Online course with video demonstrations and downloadable guides
- **Overview:** Covers equipment usage, procedural best practices, and patient-specific considerations for tracheostomy care in the home setting.
- **Ideal for:** Home health nurses aiming to enhance their tracheostomy care competencies.
- **More information:** Medbridge

3. Relias Academy – Performing Tracheostomy Care

- **Format:** Online course
- **Overview:** Focuses on familiarizing nursing professionals with tracheostomy care procedures and complication prevention in post-acute settings.
- **Ideal for:** Nurses in homecare and post-acute care environments.
- **More information:** Relias Academy

4. Clinical Skills Academy – Tracheostomy Care Training

- **Format:** Blended learning (theoretical and practical sessions)
- **Overview:** Offers a half-day course led by experienced RNs, covering tracheostomy care best practices, including suctioning, stoma care, and emergency management.
- **Ideal for:** Healthcare professionals seeking hands-on training in tracheostomy care.
- **More information:** Wren Healthcare

5. Florida Training Center – Tracheostomy Care Course

- **Format:** Online continuing education course
- **Overview:** Provides comprehensive training on tracheostomy care procedures, suitable for medical professionals seeking CE credits.
- **Ideal for:** Nurses in Florida or those looking for accredited CE courses.
- **More information:** floridatrainingcenter.org

6. BrightStar Care – Trach and Vent Care Training

- **Format:** In-house training programs
- **Overview:** Offers specialized training for healthcare providers in tracheostomy and ventilator care, emphasizing patient safety and quality of life.
- **Ideal for:** Nurses employed by or seeking employment with BrightStar Care.
- **More information:** BrightStar Care

7. Olidia Academy – Basic Tracheostomy Course

- **Format:** In-person and online courses
- **Overview:** Introduces general tracheostomy tube concepts, airway clearance, and basic respiratory equipment training.
- **Ideal for:** Nurses and caregivers entering the field of tracheostomy care.
- **More information:** olidiaacademy.com

These courses are designed to equip homecare nurses with the necessary skills and knowledge to provide safe and effective tracheostomy care. It's advisable to check with your employer or state nursing board to ensure the selected course meets any specific requirements or standards.

For pediatric homecare nurses, comfort, durability, and mobility are key when it comes to uniforms and shoes—especially when working long shifts in clients' homes where you may be on the floor, lifting, or crouching.

Here are some top recommendations for comfortable nursing uniforms and shoes:

👚 Comfortable Nursing Uniforms (Scrubs) for Homecare Nurses

1. FIGS

- **Pros**: Lightweight, stretchy, wrinkle-resistant, modern fit
- **Recommended Line:** Yola skinny scrub pants + Catarina top
- **Why it's great for homecare:** Professional yet super comfy for long wear, especially when moving around or assisting pediatric patients on the floor.

2. Cherokee Infinity

- **Pros:** Moisture-wicking, antimicrobial fabric, flexible
- **Recommended Line:** Infinity Mock Wrap Top + Jogger Scrub Pants
- **Bonus:** Deep pockets for supplies—perfect for home visits.

3. Grey's Anatomy by Barco

- **Pros:** Buttery soft, classic fit, wrinkle-resistant
- **Recommended Line:** Signature series for a clean look and comfort
- **Why it's great:** Ideal for both day and night shifts; stylish but practical.

4. Jaanuu

- **Pros:** Stretchy, antimicrobial, fashion-forward
- **Recommended Line:** 4-pocket joggers and ribbed-neck scrub top
- **Why homecare nurses love them:** Durable in various environments, including homes with pets or kids.

Comfortable Shoes for Homecare Nurses

1. HOKA One One Bondi or Clifton

- **Pros:** Maximum cushioning, podiatrist-recommended
- **Why great:** Excellent for nurses on their feet all day—good for walking, standing, and even kneeling in patients' homes.

2. Brooks Ghost or Glycerin

- **Pros:** Excellent support, slip-resistant, soft soles
- **Why nurses choose them:** Great for indoor/outdoor wear, supportive during long shifts.

3. Dansko XP 2.0 Clogs

- **Pros:** Supportive arch, slip-resistant, easy to clean
- **Best for:** Nurses who prefer clogs with orthopedic support.

4. New Balance 990 Series

- **Pros:** Durable, breathable, and offers solid ankle and heel support

- **Why it's good:** Comfort meets long-wear performance—perfect for 12-hour shifts.

5. Skechers Work Sure Track or Arch Fit

- **Pros:** Budget-friendly, memory foam, slip-resistant
- **Good for:** Nurses who want good comfort at a lower price point.
- 🧦 **Pro Tip:** Don't forget compression socks!

Reduces fatigue and swelling, especially important for day or night shift nurses doing 12 hours or more.

Here's a printable checklist PDF style breakdown for:

✅ Comfortable Nursing Uniforms & Shoes Checklist for Homecare Nurses

For both Day & Night Shifts

Title: Shift by Shift Essentials

👚 Nursing Scrubs (Uniforms)

	Brand / Item	Features	Notes
☐	FIGS (Catarina Top + Yola Pant)	Stretchy, wrinkle-free, sleek fit	Stylish & functional
☐	Cherokee Infinity	Antimicrobial, moisture-wicking, flexible	Great for hot weather
☐	Grey's Anatomy (Signature Line)	Ultra-soft, professional look	Feels like pajamas!
☐	Jaanuu	Antimicrobial, stylish, structured fit	Breathable and modern

👟 Shoes for Nurses on the Go

	Brand / Item	Features	Notes
☐	HOKA One One (Bondi or Clifton)	Ultra-cushioned, podiatrist-approved	Best for high activity
☐	Brooks (Ghost or Glycerin)	Soft soles, excellent arch support	Ideal for long days
☐	Dansko XP 2.0 Clogs	Orthopedic support, slip-resistant	Best for standing work
☐	New Balance 990 Series	Sturdy, all-day comfort	Durable indoors & outdoors
☐	Skechers Work or Arch Fit	Affordable, slip-resistant, memory foam	Budget-friendly pick

🧦 Extras

	Item	Purpose	Notes
☐	Compression Socks	Reduces swelling, boosts circulation	Must-have for long shifts
☐	Underscrub Layer (Long Sleeve)	Keeps warm in cold homes	Pick breathable fabric
☐	Extra Scrub Set	Backup for soiling or spills	Leave one in car or bag

References

American Association for Respiratory Care (AARC). (n.d.). AARC Continuing Education and Certification.

Retrieved from https://www.aarc.org

BAYADA Home Health Care. (n.d.). Homecare University: Pediatric Homecare.

Retrieved from https://www.bayada.com

Breathe California. (n.d.). Ventilator and Tracheostomy Care Training.

Retrieved from https://www.breathecalifornia.org

Infusion Nurses Society (INS). (n.d.). Feeding Tube Management and G-Tube Care.

Retrieved from https://www.ins1.org

Lincare. (n.d.). Respiratory Therapy and Care for Ventilator and Tracheostomy Patients.

Retrieved from https://www.lincare.com

National Association for Homecare & Hospice (NAHC). (n.d.). Home Health Care Training and Certification.

Retrieved from https://www.nahc.org

National Tracheostomy Safety Project. (n.d.). Tracheostomy Safety and Care Resources.

Retrieved from https://www.tracheostomy.com

Pediatric Home Service. (n.d.). Pediatric Tracheostomy and Ventilator Care Training.

Retrieved from https://www.pediatrichomeservice.com

The American Lung Association. (n.d.). Tracheostomy and Respiratory Care Education.

Retrieved from https://www.lung.org

Ventilator-Assisted Children's Home Program (VACH). (n.d.). Ventilator and Tracheostomy Care for Children.

Retrieved from https://www.choc.org

Books and Journal Articles:

Author, A. A. (Year). Title of Book. Edition (if applicable). Publisher.

Author, B. B. (Year). "Title of Article". Journal Name, Volume(Issue), Page numbers. DOI/Publisher.

www.ingramcontent.com/pod-product-compliance
Lightning Source LLC
LaVergne TN
LVHW051129210926
848482LV00001B/29
* 9 7 9 8 3 4 9 5 6 4 0 3 1 *